Healing Foods:

Prevent and Treat Common Illnesses with Fruits, Vegetables, Herbs, and More

Healing Foods:

Prevent and Treat Common Illnesses with Fruits, Vegetables, Herbs, and More

Dale Pinnock

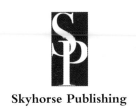

Skyhorse Publishing

Skyhorse Publishing books may be purchased in bulk at special discounts
for sales promotion, corporate gifts, fund-raising, or educational purposes.
Special editions can also be created to specifications.
For details, contact the Special Sales Department, Skyhorse Publishing,
307 West 36th Street, 11th Floor, New York, NY 10018 or
info@skyhorsepublishing.com.

www.skyhorsepublishing.com

10 9 8 7 6 5 4 3 2 1

Library of Congress Cataloging-in-Publication Data

Pinnock, Dale, 1977-
Healing Foods: Prevent and Treat Common Illnesses with Fruits,
Vegetables, Herbs, and More / Dale Pinnock.
p. cm.
Includes index.
ISBN 978-1-61608-298-7 (pbk. : alk. paper)
1. Functional foods. 2. Diet therapy. 3. Materia medica, Vegetable. I. Title.
QP144.F85P56 2011
613.2—dc22
2010044132

Printed in Italy by Rotolito Lombarda

Picture Credits
John Garon : p.2, p.104, p.109 / **Visipix.com:** p.4 / **Rocky Mountain Laboratories, NIAID, NIH:**
p. 31 / **US Department of Health - CDC - Dr. Mae Melvin:** p.73 / **All other pictures under Creative
Commons License with attribution to:** calebkimbrough: p. 13; s13610: p. 15; SqueakyMarmot: p. 18;
julie@organikal: p. 21; dmswart: p. 25; Scoro: p. 34; Schilling 2: p. 37; shimgray: p. 39; mckaysavage: p.41;
seelensturm: p.44; shioshvili: p. 47; JMRosenfeld: p.52; Vvillamon: p.55; Jude Doyland: p.59; smleon: p.61; Andrew
Michaels: p. 65; Mavis: p. 71; felipe_gabaldon: p.78; FotoosVanRobin: p. 80, p. 147, p.153; David Davies: p. 84;
smoorenburg: p. 87; xJasonRogersx: p. 96; yanivba: p. 98; theseanster93: p.100; Hari Prasad Nadig: p. 108;
quinn.anya: p.116; dotbenjamin: p.118; Jeen Na: p.123; Muffet: p.126; Andrew Morrell Photography: p.129;
lovejanine: p. 131; Arria Belli: p.136; king_david_uk: p.140; YimHafiz: p.142; mfdudu: p.157; larryjh1234: p.158;
Bill Hails: p.160; Jeff Kubina: p.163; izik: p.165; heathervescent: p.169; Skånska Matupplevelser: p.170; JACoulter:
p.173; SweetOnVeg: p.177; Clearly Ambiguous: p.181; Charleston's TheDigitel: p.183.

Contents

Thank you

Jenny Liddle – your tireless hard work and belief in me has moved mountains in the last 12 months – watch out World!! Tanya Murkett – for being a nonstop source of inspiration in every day of my life, and bringing light when all around is dark. I'd have no idea where I would be, a single day without you! Nick Salt – your wisdom, support, and insight have shaped my life immeasurably. Mum and Dad, Cheryl Thallon, Ramsay and Candy, Judith and co at Right Way, Shazzie, all the Westminster University survivors. The myriads of people who have enjoyed my work and sent me so many lovely messages – you are the reason I do this. All the regulars to my radio shows, and subscribers to my website – you are the greatest!

1

A New Paradigm in Food

●

OUR ATTITUDES to food aren't what they used to be. That's certainly true. Not so long ago, here in the UK, the 'meat and two veg' approach was the norm in most households. Many of us would see our food as simply fuel, to keep us going through the day. Something just to fill us up and give us energy. The more we ate, the stronger we became, or so we thought, and many of us would leave the house, ready to take on the day, having eaten a full breakfast.

Today, we have finally started to make the connection between food and our health. No more do we see food as just a bit of bulky fuel. Modern science has proved unequivocally that the food we eat has a direct impact upon our health and wellbeing. By making the right dietary choices, we can essentially trigger, or prevent, disease.

With such realizations in mind, modern science has started to delve deeper into the world of what we eat. Foods are being analyzed down to their most basic of components, and are revealing all manner of secrets. The actions of different nutrients on body systems are being studied in the context of disease management, and the links between nutrient deficiency and increased disease states are getting stronger as each month goes by.

The public is also more informed than ever before, and healthy food is "big" in the media. Every day new articles abound that tell us what foods are good for us and why, and what to avoid and why. There are new snippets of information about what is thought to be the next superfood, or the next food that has been linked with cancer, or the next food to make you look twenty years younger. While some of this information may be faddy and not always accurate, it has certainly created a buzz around food. It has made eating healthily something that's actually quite cool and sociable. It has made us think in a different way about what we put in our mouths, and opened up a whole wonderful world of new possibilities, not only in what we can create in the kitchen, but also in the levels to which we can take our health.

We now have an incredible wealth of information at our fingertips. My aim in this book is to convey some of this knowledge, in a new and exciting way, to inspire you and to show you how easy and enjoyable eating for health can be.

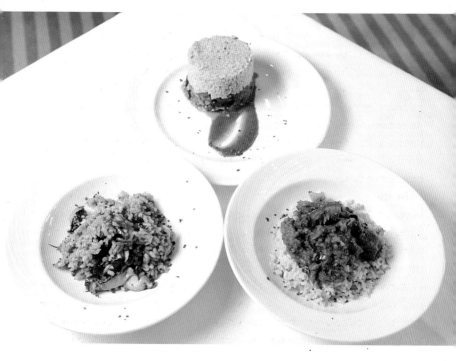

2
Food and Medicine – No Separation

●

HIPPOCRATES, the father of modern medicine, famously once said, "Let food be thy medicine, and thy medicine be thy food." Every recorded healing system on the planet, through every conceivable historical age, has recognized the vitally important role that food has to play in both maintaining good health and, indeed, turning around disease patterns. Many ancient cultures relied purely upon food remedies as their source of medicine, and many, such as Ayurveda and Traditional Chinese Medicine, studied the intricate relationships between food and physiological functions for millennia. Often, they used terms that relate to supposed "energetic" patterns and activities in foods, and how these would interplay with similar energetic patterns and events in the body, to either cause balance or harm.

In the last two centuries, the study surrounding the relationship between food, our body, and our health has been moving at quite a pace. Quite early on, we discovered things such as proteins and carbohydrates, realizing their importance in energy production and tissue maintenance. Piece by piece, we became aware of the individual vitamins and the physiological roles that they played. We became all too aware of the negative consequences of being deficient in these vital compounds, but there was seldom research that focused on the potential of these compounds to actively heal the body. As nutritional

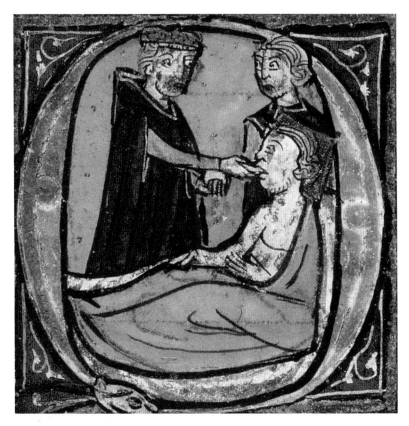

Hippocrates Medicating a Patient

science progressed, we focused on things such as the calorie, saturated and unsaturated fats, and body mass index (BMI). Nutritional science now has reached a bit of a sticking point. The dieticians may well tell you that we know all there is to know, and that eating x amount of calories will keep you at a healthy weight, and that at a certain weight and height you need y amount of a specific vitamin or nutrient.

The truth is that food's impact upon our health is enormous. It goes far beyond simply counting calories and eating our greens. Nutrition alone serves more than a maintenance role. Nutrients, vitamins, and minerals are all cofactors. This means that they directly influence the activity of very specific and vital physiological events, metabolic pathways, and biochemical reactions within our bodies. To this end, a few smart individuals began to realize that the manipulation of nutrient intake can have a huge impact upon both the severity and the progression of disease. This is because it can directly manipulate the internal biochemical terrain. It comes down to the key philosophy that underpins all natural medicine and natural healthcare. That is, the body has its own inherent ability to heal itself when given the right environment. We, as practitioners of natural healthcare, merely facilitate that correct environment.

Let's use the example of a cut on your finger. After a few minutes, the bleeding stops. Within a few hours, a scab has formed, and the body is well under way at repairing the damaged tissue. Now, if we were to continually pick at the scab, it would cause the wound to bleed and prevent healing from taking place. Well, eating a diet that consists of processed junk food, full of toxic additives, and devoid of nutrients, is the equivalent of picking at that scab. But, if we are consuming a diet of fresh, wholesome, unadulterated ingredients, we are, in fact, creating an environment that is conducive to healing.

To illustrate the above, let's look at dietary fats. Whatever you may believe, fats are a vital part of the human diet. However, we need the right ones. The fats that we consume can have a massive impact upon both the initiation of disease and the body's own ability to manage it. When we metabolize (chemically process, following digestion and absorption) certain fats, our body produces a series of biochemical messengers called *prostaglandins*. These complex molecules, among other things, are actually involved in either the instigation and enhancement of pain and inflammation, or the prevention and reduction of pain and inflammation, depending on which type is produced. The type of prostaglandins that are produced can be greatly influenced by the type of dietary fats we consume. If we eat predominantly fats that fall into the omega 3, polyunsaturated fat category, then we will direct our bodies to make a far higher percentage of the type of prostaglandins that help to reduce inflammation and minimize pain. However, if we tend to eat more saturated animal fats, then we direct our bodies to manufacture more of the prostaglandins that instigate and enhance pain and inflammation. It is obvious to see that increasing inflammation can worsen and even trigger certain conditions and complications, whereas if we are able to reduce inflammation, it is just as obvious that we can greatly benefit many conditions.

This is a miniscule glance at the influence that dietary changes can have on our internal environment in a way that can help to manage disease. For this reason, I personally feel that there is no separation between food and medicine at all. If applied in the right way under the right guidance, the results can be equally as powerful.

All of the above refers to the study of nutrition, and what we know about the way in which nutrients actually interact with our bodies and the healing potential that nutrition can hold. However, the staggering results that we observe when people drastically change their diet, focusing on minimally processed plant foods, far exceed the physical changes that we would expect to see from merely increasing our nutritional profile. There are other elements present in these foods that act as incredibly powerful medicines. These hidden magic bullets are revealed in the next chapter...

3
Phytochemicals – The Pharmacy in our Food

●

Phyto = plant.

A S MANY OF US are aware, food has the ability to drastically harm or profoundly heal. Simple changes in diet can have almost miraculous powers in the healing of many disorders. Skin conditions, inflammatory diseases, digestive ailments, low immunity, all respond rapidly from dietary interventions.

A huge amount of research and scientific investigation has focused upon nutrition as a healing modality. The role of every conceivable nutrient has now been studied in the context of prevention and disease management. We are aware of the way in which every nutrient interacts with metabolic functions and biochemical pathways, in a way that can influence specific biochemical outcomes. We know the clinical implications of low levels of certain nutrients, and we have theorized many ways in which to address this in the clinical setting. However, it seems that focusing on purely the nutritional element of food always seems to fall short. The use of nutritional supplements never delivers the same level of healing and transformation as occurs when a complete dietary overhaul is undertaken (although, in my clinics I often use a combination of both dietary change and supplementation). The reason for this is simple. Nutrition is just one part of an incredibly broad, complex, and wondrous picture. Why is this? Because fresh food contains a whole cocktail of substances that reach so far beyond the scope of nutrition alone. These substances are the phytochemicals.

The realizations that I came to at different stages of my career led me to unlock the secrets that food hold. The initial stages of this began in the late 1990s. I began experimenting with my health as a teenager. I tried every supplement, exercise programme, and diet you could imagine. The only thing that ever really caused a huge shift in my health was a diet focused around fresh plant foods. Whenever I went back to a diet that was more like the typical Western diet, but accompanied by a whole cocktail of nutritional supplements, I would start feeling awful, and the benefits I had once experienced began to decline. From the nutritional perspective, I was taking in a level of nutrients that should, according to all of the supplement gurus, leave me feeling super human. But no! Something was missing, and I knew it was more than nutrition alone. During my nutrition studies, I thought I might find the answer, but sadly didn't. We spoke about weird arbitrary terms like BMI, and measuring calories and fat. It wasn't until I began my degree in Herbal Medicine at London's University of Westminster that the penny finally dropped, and I suddenly made sense of what fresh food was delivering that supplements did not.

One of the main areas of focus in the study of Herbal Medicine is plant biochemistry and how this interacts with human physiological systems in order to bring about changes conducive to healing and correct functioning again. It was basically applied phytochemistry. Pharmacologists and pharmacognosists (people who study the medicinal chemistry of plants) unlocked the biochemical secrets that made the healing plants of ancient texts clearly valid in the modern scientific world. Suddenly it dawned on me. I knew that there were many very dull and dry texts out there that showed a full biochemical breakdown of individual foods. The search began. After a while, it became completely obvious that many of the actual pharmacologically active chemicals that are found in medicinal plants, that actually make them medicinal, are also present in notable concentrations in culinary plants. That had to be the answer. When we consume a diet that centres mostly on fresh plant foods, we are wading through nature's potent medicine cabinet. We are consuming a vast quantity of chemical compounds that deliver some incredible healing actions. These compounds aren't nutrients at all, because they are not *vital* for normal functioning. What they are is nature's potent medicinal bonus. They are pharmacologically active medicines!

So why are they there?

Phytochemicals play a myriad of different functions in plants. Some may be vivid striking colour pigments, like the deep purple *betacyanin* found in beetroot. Others may serve a hormone-like function in the plant or regulate different stages of the plant's growth. Others may become part of the plant's structure or act as a readily available food source for the plant.

What can they do for us?

The actions of phytochemicals in the body are as varied as the number of phytochemicals found in nature. They can help manage inflammation, activate enzyme systems, influence hormone systems, to name but a few activities. Below are some examples of well known phytochemicals and the activities that they deliver.

Allicin – is a powerful and pungent sulphurous chemical found in garlic, one of the things responsible for its powerful pong. Allicin is known to be a powerful antibacterial and antiviral agent. It is also known to be a circulatory stimulant and powerful antioxidant.

Anthocyanins – are deep purple/red colour pigments, such as those found in blueberries, grapes, and red onions. These pigments are powerful anti-inflammatories and are known to protect the inner lining of arteries, helping protect them from rupture that will lead to heart attack or stroke. They are also known to relax blood vessel walls a little, thus lowering blood pressure.

Beta Glucans – are very complex, heavyweight sugar compounds that are found in structural elements of seeds and fungi. These potent compounds are one of the most powerful influential forces upon human immunity. They can drastically stimulate the production of white blood cells and make them act far more aggressively when they come into contact with invaders. They are proving to be great at regulating immune responses too. Recent research carried out at the Breakspear Hospital in the UK suggests that these compounds may prove a valuable treatment for auto-immune conditions. Beta glucans also are known to have a very powerful cholesterol-lowering action.

Coumarins – these compounds play many roles in plants. They regulate root growth, cell elongation in stems, leaf thickening, and inhibit the germination of seeds. These chemicals are very aromatic. They give the distinctive smell to celery and are also the chemicals that fragrance the air when a lawn is being mown. In the body, coumarins are of great benefit to the lymphatic system. This is the filtration system of all body tissues. Coumarins actually cause a contraction of lymphatic vessels, helping lymphatic fluid to circulate and carry the toxic waste it has collected to the liver and kidneys for breakdown and removal.

The above is by no means an exhaustive list. There are literally thousands of active phytochemicals that we are aware of that can have a powerful medicinal effect upon our bodies, and these are going to be explored in all of the recipes that I have created for this book. Welcome to this beautiful and complex gift from the natural world.

4

Medicinal Cookery – System by System

●

THE BEAUTY OF understanding phytochemistry, and how nature offers us a delicious pharmacy, is that we can create an abundance of medicinal morsels from the simplest of ingredients. When we understand what foods contain what chemicals, and how these chemical compounds influence our body's chemistry in order to deliver a healing response, we can get into the kitchen and cook up and create our own medicine.

About the Recipes

Take care when handling chillies, and remember to wash your hands thoroughly after touching them.

The Skin

Our skin is the largest organ in our body. Many of us don't see it as an organ, but that's exactly what it is. Apart from the obvious function of being a barrier between the outside world and the soft delicate tissues within our body, our skin has some vital regulatory functions. It is the first stage of immunity. In addition to the skin physically blocking pathogens from entering our body, there is also a dense bacterial population living on the outer surface of the skin which help us fight against any pathogens that may be trying their luck. The dichotomy is, however, that these bacteria, if given the opportunity, can cause infection themselves, such as that which occurs in a spot.

Our skin also plays a vital role in temperature regulation. Even the slightest changes in body temperature can be disastrous to our health. Our skin keeps us cool by allowing us to sweat. When we sweat, it rapidly helps the body to cool as the moisture evaporates off our skin. If we get too cold, the skin makes all the hairs on our body, both large and small, to stand erect. This helps to keep our body more insulated.

The other major role that our skin plays is to give us the sense of touch. Thousands of nerve endings permeate the layers of the skin, enabling us to detect even a delicate cobweb that touches our face.

Therapeutic management of skin conditions

Skin lesions can be distressing. Our skin, especially on our face, hands, and arms, is on constant display to the outside world. It is definitely one of the most personally distressing types of disorders to afflict us. In general, whatever the route cause and trigger, skin conditions always come down to two distinct factors – infection and inflammation. Acne is, of course, a prime example of both of these elements in action. When infection arises in a blocked pore, localized inflammation ensues. If we learn natural ways to manage both of these responses, we can have a huge impact upon both the appearance and future development of skin disorders.

Regulating oil production

Sebum, the natural oil found in our skin, produced in tiny glands within hair follicles, is a vital factor for skin health. It regulates moisture levels, offers protection against age-related damage, and also makes the skin waterproof. In normal circumstances, we are generally unaware that it is there. However, those with oily, acne-prone skin, or those with excessively dry skin, will be acutely aware of the impact that it can have upon the health of the skin. It is sebum that is the main cause of spot formation. If our sebum fills pores in the skin to a certain level, and is at a certain viscosity, it can begin to oxidize –

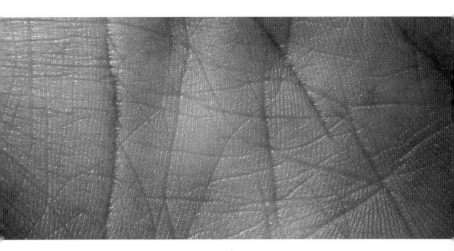

especially if it fills the pore to the extent that it can come into contact with air. When this occurs, it begins to get tough, turns a dark colour, and a comedone or "blackhead" is formed. Blackheads then become a collection site for bacteria such as staphylococcus, which live naturally and harmlessly on the outer surface of the skin. When such bacteria collect around a comedone, it eventually sets off an infection, and, hey presto, a spot forms.

There are many factors in our bodies that can affect sebum and what it does. The hormone testosterone, for example, can aggravate and drastically increase the production of sebum. Testosterone also makes the sebum far more viscous, so more likely to block the pore and cause infection.

Enhancing normal detoxification

Try to keep the internal environment of the body as clean as possible. The skin, after all, is the fourth major route of elimination for toxic waste. When our body processes toxic material, to make it ready for removal from the body, it will usually send it in one of two directions for removal. If the toxic compound can be made water-soluble by the liver, it will be sent to the kidneys for removal via the urine. If it can be made fat-soluble, the liver will send it, via bile, to the bowel, to be removed that way. Waste products in the lymphatic system will also generally be sent to the kidneys. Some toxins are volatile, meaning they will evaporate easily. Such compounds will be removed from the body via the breath. If these normal routes of elimination get over-burdened (which, let's face it, isn't difficult in the modern world), one of the first things the body will do is send toxic matter to the skin for rapid removal. When this happens, the skin appears in worse condition, lesions take longer to heal, and there is more toxic material present to potentially aggravate the skin. Therefore, to help your skin to heal, it's important to eat foods and follow practices that enhance normal detoxification mechanisms.

Regulating inflammation
Almost all skin lesions, regardless of their cause, involve inflammation. Eczema is a perfect example of an inflammatory condition. It is what we call a type 2 hypersensitivity reaction. This basically means that the body's own immune system has become overly sensitized to a specific stimulus. This could be a food, or something in the local environment such as a detergent or pollutant. Whenever the immune system comes into contact with this specific stimulus, it delivers a normal immunological response, but in a far more aggressive way than is necessary. This then causes inflammation in the upper layers of the skin, and the typical eczema lesion, of raised, red, itchy patches ensues.

There are many foods that can help the body to reduce its inflammatory load. Many of these foods interrupt normal chemical reactions that switch inflammation on. Others actually manipulate the production of biochemicals that regulate the rate and extent of inflammation in the body.

Omega Butter Crostinis

SERVES 1

This amazing dish is like a super-charged version of peanut butter on toast. It makes an incredible breakfast, and is a nutritional and medicinal explosion.

2 handfuls of pumpkin seeds
2 handfuls of sunflower seeds
1 handful of hemp seeds
3 tablespoons flaxseed oil
1 teaspoon sea salt

1. Add all the ingredients to a food processor and blend into a smooth butter.
2. Serve on toasted wholegrain bread.

MEDICINAL PROPERTIES

Pumpkin Seeds – are a real powerhouse. They contain huge amounts of naturally occurring zinc. This vital nutrient plays a significant role in the treatment of acne. Zinc is involved in the regulation of many hormonal systems in the body, not to mention controlling certain functions within the immune system which will directly affect the healing time of wounds.

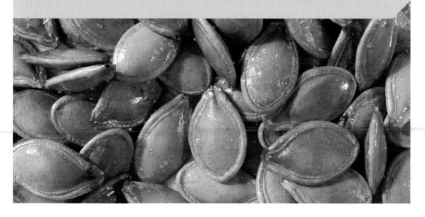

Zinc also regulates the activity of the sebaceous glands, helping to keep excessive oil production to a minimum. In addition, it reduces the way in which testosterone affects the production of keratin and sebum, keeping initial spot formation to a minimum.

There is also a compound present in pumpkin seeds called *beta sitosterol*, which is thought to make testosterone behave in a far less aggressive manner. Many people, therefore, believe that it may also give added benefit to acne sufferers, especially to boys.

Pumpkin seeds are also incredibly rich in both omega 3 and omega 6 essential fatty acids, which help to greatly reduce the impact of the inflammatory process. The redness associated with spots is the inflammatory process in action. Omega 3 fatty acids actually provide the building blocks for the body to manufacture its own natural anti-inflammatory compounds – series 1 and 3 prostaglandins. Increasing the body's natural production of these compounds can notably reduce the appearance of redness, making spots look far less affected than they are. This will also speed up healing time.

Sunflower Seeds – are very similar to pumpkin seeds, from the nutritional perspective. They are very dense in zinc. They differ from pumpkin seeds in that they seem to house a much more powerful anti-inflammatory activity. They have been used in this context for centuries in folk medicine. Many believe that this anti-inflammatory activity is due to the fatty acid content of the seeds. However, the anti-inflammatory activity displayed by sunflower seeds, in relation to the actual levels of these fats, is far greater than can be explained by merely the fats alone. This suggests that there is something else present in these seeds that is responsible that still currently eludes discovery.

Hemp Seeds – are another fatty acid powerhouse. Hemp contains a very high quality source of omega 6 fatty acids. These play a vital role in skin health, as they help control water loss through the skin. This greatly affects moisture balance in the skin, which can drastically alter the overall appearance of the skin, making any lesions or outbreaks appear worse.

Classic Carrot and Ginger Soup

SERVES 4

This recipe is an absolute classic and a real winter warmer. It is wonderful for anyone fighting a skin disorder, as it offers tremendous support from both a nutritional and a medicinal perspective.

5 large carrots
1 baking potato
2 sticks of celery
5 cm (2 inch) piece of ginger
2 cloves of garlic
1 red onion
Vegetable stock

1. Coarsely chop the carrots and potato, leaving the skins on both. Finely slice the celery. Finely chop the ginger, the garlic, and the onion.
2. In a pan, sauté the ginger, garlic, celery, and onion, along with a pinch of crystal salt, until the onion is softened.
3. At this stage, add the chopped carrot and potato, and add enough vegetable stock to just cover the vegetables. Simmer until the vegetables are almost soft, then blend into a smooth, bright orange soup.

MEDICINAL PROPERTIES

Carrots – are skin food through and through. The bright orange colour pigment in carrots is due to the presence of beta carotene. This pigment is also the plant source of vitamin A. This is a vital nutrient for skin health. Firstly, beta carotene plays a role in the activity of sebaceous glands, regulating how much oil they produce, and at what rate it is produced.

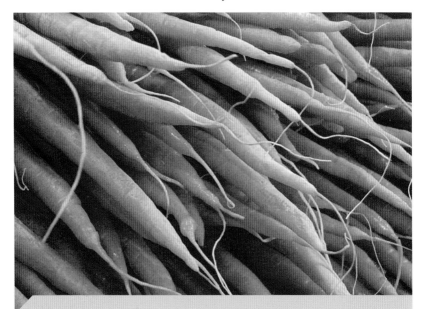

Secondly, beta carotene is known to protect the skin against UV damage, and to help repair damage. This gives skin a better appearance in the long run.

Beta carotene also has some notable anti-inflammatory effects, and regular consumption of dietary carotenoids can help to minimize inflammation.

Celery – is a great all-round detoxifier and cleanser. This is because it contains a group of chemicals called *coumarins*. These are the same compounds that fill the air with aroma when a lawn is mown. Coumarins stimulate the lymphatic system, encouraging a contraction of lymphatic vessel walls, which in turn increases circulation of lymphatic fluid, ready for removal of waste products at the relevant places. So what is the implication of this for the skin? Well, the lymphatic system is essentially the filtration system of all body tissues. It helps to carry away waste products and toxins, sending them for removal via the liver and kidneys. Stimulating this system to work at its best will enhance the rate at which toxins and waste products are removed from the skin. This will help keep the skin clearer, make it appear brighter and healthier, and also increase healing time.

Onion – is a very rich source of the mineral sulphur, which is absolutely vital for the health of the skin. Sulphur helps maintain the proteins that give skin its structure, making onions an important food for skin health and improved overall appearance of skin.

Onions are also a rich source of a compound called *quercetin*. This flavonoid compound that is associated with colour pigments in plants is known to be a very powerful anti-inflammatory agent, so can help to reduce redness of skin lesions.

Ginger – could be described as "the king of anti-inflammatory foods". The powerful essential oils that give ginger its spicy taste and aroma form part of a very complex inflammation-busting chemistry. Ginger is useful for any inflammatory problem in the body, and can play a really important part in the management of any skin condition. As most of the common skin conditions, from eczema and psoriasis, through to acne, involve inflammation, ginger should become a regular food in your diet.

Chickpea, Squash, and Rainbow Chard Curry

SERVES 4

Serve with a side salad.

2 cloves of garlic, finely chopped
1 red onion, finely chopped
2.5 cm (1 inch) piece of fresh ginger, peeled and finely chopped
2 tablespoons Thai green curry paste
250 g (9 oz) butternut squash, cubed
1 can (14 oz/400 g size) cooked chickpeas
1 heaped tablespoon peanut butter
10 fl oz (300 ml/1¼ cups) coconut milk
4 fl oz (120 ml/½ cup) vegetable stock
2 large bunches of rainbow chard, shredded

1. Add the garlic, onion, and ginger to a pan with a little oil, and begin to sauté until the onion starts to turn a lighter colour.
2. At this stage add the curry paste, and continue to sauté until the whole mixture becomes highly fragrant.
3. Add the squash, chickpeas, and peanut butter, and mix well.
4. Add the coconut milk and the stock. Simmer gently for about 30 minutes, until the squash becomes tender.
5. Add in the rainbow chard until it wilts. The curry is ready to serve.

MEDICINAL PROPERTIES

Chickpeas – are one of my absolute staples. I can't get enough of them! From the bare bones' nutritional perspective, they are very high fibre, which helps to clear waste out of the digestive tract. This in itself can give the skin an extra glow. They are also very high in zinc, so can be a good aid to skin healing.

Chickpeas are also rich in a rare trace mineral called *molybdenum*, which among other things can assist in the breakdown of certain environmental and metabolic toxins in the liver.

Butternut Squash – is a delicious anti-inflammatory food. Its rich orange flesh is bursting with the plant pigment beta carotene, such as that found in carrots. This delivers powerful anti-inflammatory activity. It also supplies a huge boost in vitamin A, which helps to regulate oil production in the skin, and give the skin a more youthful appearance.

Rainbow Chard – is a very close relative of the humble beetroot. As such, it contains a good level of a compound called *betacyanin*, which is the red pigment found in the stems and veins of these delicious leaves. Betacyanin is known to speed up certain functions within the liver that break down toxic matter and prepare it for removal from the body. This particular function is a series of chemical processes known as "phase 2 detoxification", which is the second stage of processing that the liver uses before sending processed toxins to either the kidneys or bowel. Enhancing such processes can help the skin in the long run, as it keeps the levels of toxic waste down.

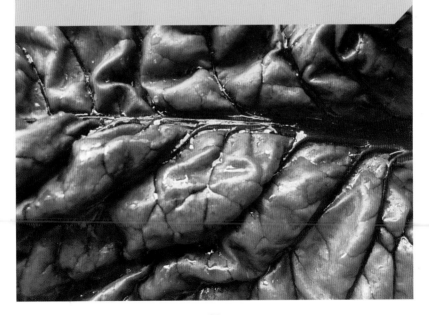

Artichoke, Red Onion, Spinach and Black Olive Dairy-free Pizza

SERVES 1

Yes, you are still reading the same book. Pizza doesn't need to be the greasy, over priced cheese on toast that we associate with being hideously bad for us. If made in the right way, pizza can be a filling and healthy dinner. This one in particular is absolute heaven, and full of ingredients that are beneficial to many body systems, not just the skin.

150 g (5½ oz) plain wholemeal flour
1 teaspoon baking powder
2 tablespoons passata (sieved tomatoes)
1 clove of garlic, finely chopped
¼ red onion, diced
1 handful of spinach, steamed or wilted
5–6 pieces of marinated artichoke hearts
1 tablespoon pitted black olives

1. Preheat the oven to 220°C/425°F/Gas mark 7. In a bowl, mix the flour and baking powder together. Start adding a little water to this, bit by bit. Add enough to make a stiff dough. Make sure your dough isn't soggy. Kneed by hand for about a minute, then roll out to form a very thin (half a cm maximum) pizza base.

2. Place this on a baking tray and put into the hot oven for about 3–5 minutes, until it begins to firm and take on a bread-like texture. At this point, take out of the oven. Turn the oven temperature down to 190°C/375°F/Gas mark 5.

3. Spread out the passata on the base. Add the chopped garlic and diced onion, along with a pinch of crystal salt and some ground black pepper. Layer on the wilted spinach, then the artichokes, then finally the black olives.

4. Place the pizza back into the medium hot oven, and bake until the base has firmed up and resembles a wholemeal pitta bread in texture. If you really can't live without dairy on this dish, crumble over a little goat's cheese or feta.

MEDICINAL PROPERTIES

Tomatoes (Passata) – are very rich in a powerful antioxidant phytochemical called *lycopene*. This chemical can help to protect the skin from sun damage. More importantly, it can help to reduce inflammation. Most skin lesions involve localized inflammation caused by immunological activity taking place in the area. A wide variety of potent dietary anti-inflammatories can help to minimize redness associated with such inflammatory lesions.

Artichoke – is a very powerful liver cleanser. It contains a compound called *caffeoylquinic acid*, which actually helps to stimulate the flow of bile from the liver. Bile is a transport medium that the liver uses to carry fat-soluble toxins away for removal via the bowel. The faster this occurs, the faster these toxins are removed from the body. This will certainly help the skin, as it can all too easily be used as an outlet for removing toxins, which can worsen many skin conditions.

Spinach – is a great source of beta carotene, which is the plant form of vitamin A. This vital nutrient helps to regulate oil production in the skin, and also works as an anti-inflammatory.

▶ Top Ingredients for Skin Health

Artichokes – help detoxify the liver, giving the skin a helping hand.
Butternut Squash – rich in beta carotene, helps to regulate oil production and collagen production.
Celery – keeps the lymphatic system clean and helps to detoxify.
Onion – is rich in sulphur and the anti-inflammatory chemical quercetin.
Seeds (Pumpkin, Sesame, Sunflower, Hemp, Flax) – contain high levels of essential fatty acids such as the omegas 3, 6, and 9.

▶ General Tips for Skin Health

▶ **Stay hydrated.** We have had it drummed into us for years that we need to be drinking 6–8 glasses of water a day. This is especially necessary if you want clear, vibrant-looking skin. Staying hydrated is important to skin health for two main reasons. Firstly, a hydrated skin has fewer fine lines, better elasticity, and looks generally brighter. Secondly, drinking plenty of water helps to flush out water-soluble toxins from the kidneys. Remember that the skin will be used as a fast and convenient waste removal system if any of the other modes of elimination are in any way inhibited. This can lead to skin breakouts and lesions. However, don't overdo it and drink excessive amounts of water. That can be potentially dangerous and even lead to death.

▶ **Get the best skin care possible.** A good skincare regime is essential for anyone, especially those with skin complaints. Such a regime can work wonders for the skin, and how it functions and thrives as an organ. Choose a range of products with the minimum amount of harsh chemicals. Get advice from a highly trained beauty therapist or skincare expert to find products that are best for you.

▶ **Reduce sugar intake.** OK, I know this is a hotly debated area. Many "experts" will tell you that there is no link between sugary foods and skin conditions. I personally beg to differ, and here is my reasoning. When we eat sugar, we get a very sudden rise in blood sugar. When this happens, our body initially releases adrenalin (hence the sugar rush). After a while of surging adrenalin circulating around our bodies, in an attempt to make us burn up the sugar the body will start to release insulin, in order to tell the cells to suck in the excess sugar and get it out of the bloodstream. Now, at the stage we have high levels of adrenalin in circulation, the skin is affected. Adrenalin directly stimulates the sebaceous glands in the skin. This will cause a drastic increase in the production of sebum, and increase the likelihood of developing skin 'break outs'.

▶ **Fill up on fat.** No, you aren't seeing things. I am encouraging you to eat fat. Now, before you get excited and phone the local pizza joint, I am talking about the good fats: omega 3, 6, and 9. These fats are so vital for skin health. They help to condition the skin and help to control inflammation. Plus, many of the food sources of these fats are very rich in other important nutrients such as zinc and vitamin E. Reach for sources such as hemp seeds, pumpkin seeds, algae (spirulina), and oily fish (if you are happy to eat it).

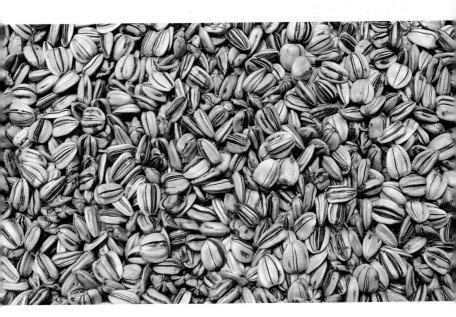

My Story

At the age of 10, things started to change. I noticed a few little bumps on my chin. Being a child, I wasn't overly concerned, as there were far more important things to worry about – fishing was my distraction of choice back then. The only thing that mattered was getting down to the lake after school and at the weekends.

A year later, it was time to wave goodbye to junior school, and head off to secondary school (high school). It was here that the trouble began. By this stage I was spotty. There's no other word for it. From forehead to chin, I was covered in nasty little red spots. It didn't take long for everyone else in the class to notice this too. As you can guess, kids being the way they are, the usual names came: Pizza face, Zit face, etc. At that stage in life, these things can make us very self-conscious and I became quite withdrawn, although I'd never let it show. By the time I reached the final year of school, it was a permanent distraction. I went to doctor after doctor, specialist after specialist, and tried every conceivable lotion and potion they had to offer. Strange sticky roll on lotions, antibiotics, retinol gels. The works. Nothing whatsoever helped.

One day, at the age of about 15–16, a friend's mum lent me a book on nutrition and natural healthcare. I remember her telling me, "Unless you look after what's going on inside, nothing will change on the outside." Now, as a teenage boy, you can imagine the type of sceptical expletives that spouted forth. However, I was desperate beyond all measure (I hated even being seen in daylight), and read the book. I read it cover to cover in a weekend, and changed everything immediately. I gave up smoking, I gave up eating meat, I gave up most dairy products, and built a diet based on fruits, vegetables, and whole grains. I supplemented with things like zinc, omega 3, and the B vitamins.

The changes were incredible. My skin certainly did clear. The red aggressive acne eventually cleared, leaving not even the slightest mark.

Beyond that, my body and mind *literally* rebuilt from the ground up, and an entirely new person was born.

I have seen the powerful effect that food can have on our health, first hand. It is simple yet profound. It was this experience that led me here today.

Digestive Problems

The digestive system is undoubtedly one of the most used and abused of body systems. Consisting of the digestive tract (the hollow tube that runs from mouth to anus), the liver, and the pancreas, the digestive system is the gateway for the abundance of beautiful foods out there to nourish us and help us grow and evolve.

Digestion starts in the mouth. Our teeth give us mechanical breakdown of large pieces of food. There are also some simple carbohydrate-digesting enzymes present in our saliva that start the process off.

The next stop is the stomach. This is a highly acidic environment that churns food round and round to assist its breakdown. The stomach is the primary location for protein digestion. Using digestive fluids such as pepsin and hydrochloric acid, proteins begin to be broken down into their individual amino-acid components. These fluids also help to kill any nasty bacteria that may have been lurking in our food.

Once our stomach has done its work, the food then gets sent on to the small intestine. The intestine is an alkaline environment, so as soon as the acidic chyme (the acidic, partially digested food stuff that leaves the stomach) enters the intestine, bile salts are released from the liver to buffer the acid, and small spurts of enzymes are released from the pancreas. The small intestine doesn't secrete any of its own digestive fluids, so relies solely on those produced by the pancreas and the liver. These enzymes help to digest dietary fats and carbohydrates, and break them down into small enough units for our body to absorb. Lining the walls of the intestine are billions of tiny finger-like projections known as villi. These little projections are porous, and absorb digested food and nutrients, and carry them in the blood to our liver. It takes about 3–5 hours for the food that leaves our stomach to become a thin, watery nutrient soup. Anything that cannot be absorbed by the villi, then makes its way to the large intestine.

The large intestine, or colon, is the final stage of the digestive journey. The watery leftovers that exit the small intestine slowly move through. As this watery mix moves through the large intestine, most of the water gets absorbed through the colon wall into the bloodstream. As this occurs, the leftover waste material gets harder and harder until a solid mass is formed – and nature's call ensues.

Therapeutic management of digestive problems

Most digestive problems share varying amounts of the same group of symptom patterns, regardless of the original cause. Obviously, the key to long-term management of digestive problems, like many physical ailments, will focus upon finding the main cause and eradicating this. However, when it comes to home remedies and food remedies, it can be vitally important to learn tips and tricks to manage symptoms, and make us feel that little bit better.

Easing gas and bloating

Gas in the digestive tract, like it or not, is a perfectly normal thing. It is caused by several factors, but the most common is an incomplete digestion of certain food stuffs. In most cases, it is specific carbohydrates that can cause the problem, especially if they are refined, heavily cooked, or eaten in close proximity to simple refined sugar. These particular carbohydrates are particularly taxing for the enzymes in the small intestine (where most digestion and absorption takes place), which leads to an incomplete breakdown and digestion of the carbs in question. Now, this can vary from individual to individual, as we are all slightly different with regard to the levels of specific enzymes we have, so a food that upsets one person may be completely fine for another. Just one of life's little nuances. When the incompletely broken down foods get to the large intestine, the good bacteria in the gut finish off the job and set to work on breaking down these food stuffs. This process causes the release of hydrogen, carbon dioxide, and, in about one third of people, methane.

While trying to figure out which foods are the most common offenders for us is the key to long-term eradication of this problem, there are thankfully some great foods that we can eat that can manage this problem naturally.

Regulating gut motility

Gut motility refers to the movement of food and waste through the entire gut. This is greatly regulated by a series of perfectly orchestrated, rhythmical contractions that move gut contents along. This rhythmical contraction is called *peristalsis*. The gut wall is lined by several layers of muscle, which contract at various times and stages, to literally squeeze the contents along. Any disruption of normal gut motility can cause havoc in our bodies. There are two main outcomes from disruption of gut motility – constipation and diarrhoea. Thankfully, with the right intervention, normal function can quickly be restored.

Constipation is a common scourge of the Western world. It essentially means that we aren't passing stools as frequently as usual. Stools can be excessively hard, difficult to pass, or we may experience incomplete emptying of the bowels. There are many causes, but the most common one is a combination of inadequate fibre intake and insufficient fluid consumed. High-fibre foods, such as fruit, vegetables, and wholegrains, all absorb a lot of water, which creates a soft, bulky stool. Refined foods, such as ready meals, white bread, white rice, etc, have very little in the way of fibre, so have little water-holding capacity, thus creating a harder stool. This gives us an idea as to how an inadequate fluid intake may affect us too. The body absorbs water through the intestine and colon. If there is little fluid available, the body will absorb as much as it physically can through the colon wall, leaving virtually nothing to soften and bulk up the stool. Drinking plenty of water, along with a high-fibre diet, allows the body to be hydrated and supplies enough to bulk up the stool.

Diarrhoea on the other hand involves excessive, spasm-like contractions that literally fire out the gut contents. This can be caused by many factors, but most commonly it is due to the presence of some mild inflammation. This could have arisen from bacterial or viral infection, food allergy, or even an auto-immune response (ulcerative colitis). The biggest risk factor associated with diarrhoea is dehydration and malnutrition, due to the food not being in the digestive tract for long enough.

Managing the 'good bacteria'

Our digestive system is a complex and flourishing eco system, awash with bacterial life. Our bodies consist of around 100 trillion cells in all. There is a staggering ten times that number of bacteria within our digestive tract – there are anywhere between 300 and 1,000 different species present there! This sounds a little alarming, but we actually have a mutually beneficial symbiotic relationship with this flora. They help us with a myriad of digestive functions, from fermenting and

Our digestive system is a complex and flourishing eco system, awash with bacterial life.

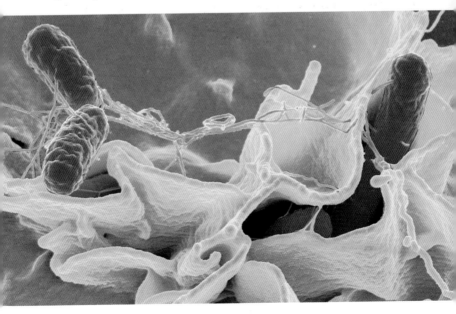

breaking down certain food groups, to regulating certain responses within the immune system, to preventing the growth of harmful bacteria. What I find to be one of the most amazing functions of gut bacteria is the healing and maintenance of the internal lining of the gut. When the gut bacteria actually ferment certain types of carbohydrate, they transform it into substances called *short chain fatty acids*, which can actually help to restore the inner lining of the digestive tract, and stimulate the growth of new cells within this lining. This can be especially important in conditions such as ulcerative colitis and intestinal permeability (aka "leaky gut").

Nothing has a greater influence on the long-term health of the gut flora than the food we eat.

Stimulating digestion

Sometimes, we can find ourselves with weakened or impaired digestion, or feeling like we have no appetite whatsoever. This can happen for a number of reasons. Illness, stress, poor diet, excessive alcohol, etc, can all cause a reduction in digestive secretions, which can leave us feeling heavy after meals, or cause us to lose any inclination to eat. Sometimes these symptoms can also be a sign of liver problems.

There are some foods that cause an increase in the production of these digestive fluids, and can really stimulate appetite and wake things up a little bit.

Digestive Tonic Tea

This simple, aromatic tea, drunk regularly, can strengthen and regulate digestive functions. It will help to regulate peristaltic contractions, increase transit time, increase the production of digestive fluids, reduce inflammation, and reduce bloating and gas.

Use equal parts of each of the following:

Peppermint
Bay leaf
Fennel seeds
Caraway seeds
Dried liquorice root

1. Blend all the dry ingredients and put in a jar as a loose tea to use daily.

2. Probably the most complex recipe I have ever written! 4 teaspoons of dry mix per cup. Add to a teapot or cafetière (French press), and allow to brew for 10 minutes. That's it!

MEDICINAL PROPERTIES

Peppermint – is a powerful digestive tonic. The essential oil menthol helps to regulate the normal rhythmical contractions of the gut wall. It can be used in both diarrhoea and constipation, because rather than slowing down or speeding up these contractions, it seems to actually regulate them in either way that they may need.

Bay Leaf – is a herb with a very long medicinal history. Once believed to be magical, this humble leaf is a very powerful carminative. This means that it helps to break down excessive gas in the digestive system and allow it to be reabsorbed by the body.

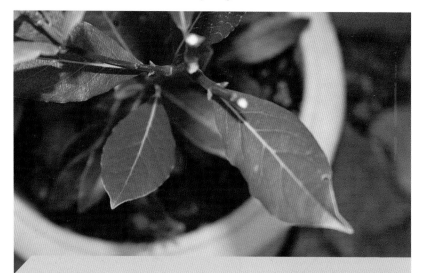

Fennel seeds – are another of nature's most powerful carminatives. Not only are they highly effective, but they are also incredibly safe and gentle. So much so that they make a fantastic tea for infant colic and griping.

Caraway seeds – are especially adept at easing painful flatulence, and are also mildly antispasmodic, so can be a great ingredient for problems such as colic and painful trapped wind.

Liquorice root – is a powerful anti-inflammatory. Many digestive complaints, such as IBS and colitis, involve a lot of inflammation. Liquorice contains a chemical called *glycyrrhetinic acid*, which works in a similar way to common steroid medications to reduce the severity of the inflammatory response, and can quite rapidly soothe swollen surfaces.

Anti-Parasite Pesto

Pesto is one of my favourite sauces. I could sit and eat a jar of it with a spoon in about a minute! This version of the classic Italian sauce is designed for people who are tackling some kind of parasitic infection in the digestive system. It blends the best anti-parasitic herbs on the planet that thankfully taste like heaven when combined.

This recipe is most successful in the treatment of *Candida albicans* infection. Candida is a simple yeast that naturally lives within our gut and commonly in the genital area. For this recipe we shall focus on its manifestation in the digestive tract. In most situations, Candida lives in a commensal manner inside us, not really causing much of a problem, and is kept in check by our population of good bacteria that police the digestive tract.

However, when environmental changes allow, Candida can start to proliferate and cause infection in the digestive tract. When it begins to take over the digestive tract, it can start to grow little tentacle-like outgrowths that can burrow through the gut wall and penetrate the blood vessels that lead from the gut – the very same vessels that contain all our precious freshly digested nutrients. These tentacles suck up our nutrients, feeding the Candida!

Now, Candida will soon get bored of sitting in one patch of gut and will quickly move on to another area close by. When it moves on, the holes left behind from its tentacles burrowing through cause the biggest problem of all. Because they are gaping holes straight into the general circulatory system, it is possible for particles of partially digested food matter to enter the bloodstream. Our body, of course, has a very sensitive and powerful immune system that can quickly recognize if there is something in the body that doesn't belong there. Because this food is only partially broken down, and not in the fully digested form that our body recognizes, the partially digested blob is treated as an invader, and our immune system mounts an attack.

The downside of this normal response happening in such unfortunate circumstances is that our body can suddenly develop an "immunity" or "immune sensitivity" to that particular food every time it is consumed, thus giving the appearance of "food allergies" that so commonly accompany Candida infection. So it is vital that this infection is dealt with promptly. Some of the symptoms associated with Candida infection are constipation, diarrhoea, headaches, fatigue, eczema, acne, psoriasis, muscle and joint pain, and even mild depression.

This sauce is a great dressing for salads, stirred raw into cooked pasta, or just eaten as a dip (which I tend to do). When prepared, this pesto will keep in the fridge for about 4 days.

3 tablespoons pumpkin seeds
1 handful of fresh basil leaves
1 clove of raw garlic
Extra virgin olive oil
Crystal salt – add to taste

This is such an easy dish to prepare. Simply place all the ingredients into a blender and blend into a smooth aromatic purée.

MEDICINAL PROPERTIES

Garlic – is without doubt one of the most profound and broad-reaching medicinal plants on the planet, and its uses and actions could fill tomes. In the context of this recipe, garlic is probably the most powerful natural anti-parasite/anti-infective agent ever discovered. This anti-infective activity is due to the powerful compound allicin. Allicin is part of the spectrum of sulphur compounds found within garlic. These are the compounds which give garlic its characteristic, pungent odour. Allicin doesn't get broken down in the digestive system, and a high percentage of it passes through the digestive tract untouched. Another small percentage is removed from the body via the lungs – hence the kiss-busting smell. It is most likely that allicin causes death of simple organisms almost on contact.

Basil – the signature herb of the Mediterranean, is another of the most powerful anti-parasitic herbs on the planet, and thankfully it tastes delicious so is no chore to consume. It is a very fragrant herb rich in powerful essential oils. These oils are the keys to its medicinal activity. These volatile oils that give basil its heavenly smell do not get broken down by the body either, and just like the compounds in garlic travel through the digestive tract and are able to blast simple organisms such as yeast, virtually on contact.

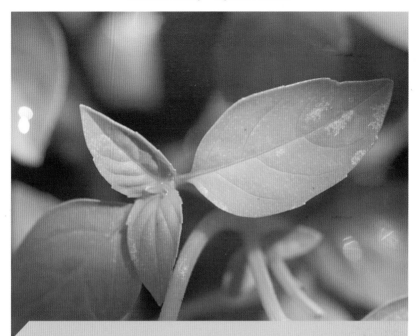

Pumpkin Seeds – replace the traditional pine nuts that are used in pesto. The addition of pumpkin seeds makes this pesto extra green. Pumpkin seeds are delicious nutritional powerhouses. They are a rich source of essential fatty acids such as omega 6 and omega 3. They are also rich in minerals, particularly zinc. However, the active constituent of interest in Candida infection is cucurbitin. Cucurbitin is a major constituent in these seeds and has shown to have a very powerful anti-parasitic effect in many test tube studies. This supports the use of these seeds by Native Americans for all manner of gastro intestinal infections. Aside from the cucurbitin, it is also believed that pumpkin seeds have a mechanical effect upon Candida, helping to literally scrape it off the intestinal walls to a certain degree. This would also be true of any high-fibre, dense foods.

Beetroot and Artichoke Quinoa Salad

SERVES 1

This is a lovely side dish. It can be eaten hot or cold, and can even be used as a stuffing for mushrooms or red peppers. It looks amazing, tastes great, and gives your liver a revamp too.

2 large handfuls of quinoa
1 small beetroot
Half a 50 g (2 oz) jar of cooked artichoke hearts
Rocket (arugula) to garnish

1. Boil the quinoa in water until it is soft, with a texture like rice.
2. Steam the beetroot until soft, then dice into small cubes.
3. Finely chop the artichoke.
4. Mix the artichoke, beetroot, and quinoa together.
5. Garnish with rocket (arugula) as a side salad.

MEDICINAL PROPERTIES

Beetroot – has a longstanding history as a powerful medicine for liver disorders. It contains a very rich, deep purple pigment called *betacyanin*. This incredibly powerful pigment helps to stimulate and enhance processes in the liver known as "phase 2 detoxification". This means that it helps the liver to process toxins such as alcohol in a much more efficient manner, to break them down faster and send them on their way for removal from the body. It is also believed that betacyanin can stimulate the production of bile, which can further aid in the removal of processed toxins.

Artichoke – contains many active chemicals, including caffeoylquinic acids, shown to speed up the production of bile in the liver, and increase the rate at which it is released from the gall bladder. Bile is the liver's natural delivery system that carries processed toxins away from the liver in order to be removed via the bowel.

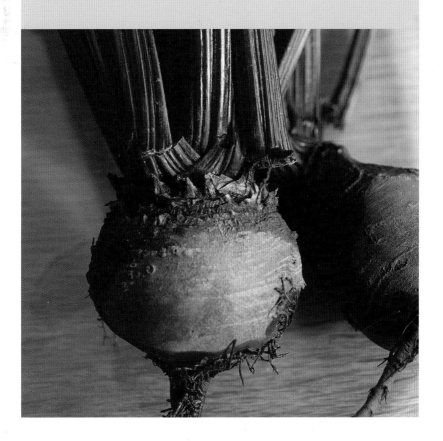

Leek, Onion, and Feta Tart, with Jerusalem Artichoke Mash

SERVES 3–4

This beautiful main meal is a creative twist on the good old British "Pie 'n Mash". It is filling, nutritionally dense, and great for encouraging the growth of good bacteria in the gut.

1 large red onion
1 large leek
1 clove of garlic
Readymade puff pastry (we all need a shortcut every now and then)
Feta cheese
4–5 Jerusalem artichokes
1 teaspoon English mustard
Salt and black pepper to taste

Preheat the oven to 180°C/350°F/Gas mark 4.

For the tart filling

Peel, and halve the red onion, and cut widthways into slices. Coarsely chop the leek into thin slices. Finely chop the clove of garlic. Add the three ingredients to a pan with a little olive oil, and a pinch of crystal salt. Sauté until the onion and leek have softened and have started to almost caramelize together. Keep to one side.

For the tart case

OK, I admit it, I usually cheat on this one and get some ready rolled puff pastry. Pastry and I don't always get along, so I find it easier. Simply roll out the pastry, to a thickness of only a few millimetres. Line a 25 cm (10 inch) tart case with it, discarding the excess. Fill the case with baking beads, or dried beans, and "blind bake" for 3–5 minutes, to enable the bottom of the case to just start to get crispy. Remove the baking beads, then add the leek and onion

40

mixture. Crumble over some Feta cheese, enough to give a light covering of the filling mixture. Bake in the oven for 15 minutes, or until the pastry rises and starts to go crisp and golden.

For the Jerusalem artichoke mash
Simply cube the Jerusalem artichokes, and boil in a pan until soft. Drain, then return to the pan with a little olive oil, and the English mustard, and mash until smooth.

To serve
Take a good slice of the tart, a few dollops of the mash, and serve with a good, colourful, mixed side salad.

MEDICINAL PROPERTIES

Onions – being a close relative of garlic have a similar chemistry and similar medicinal properties, although to a slightly lesser degree. Onions contain a fabulous compound called *inulin*, that works as a prebiotic agent. This means that it encourages the growth of good bacteria in the gut, by providing them with a food source. This helps to increase the number of the good, and decrease the number of the bad, fine-tuning digestive health when consumed regularly.

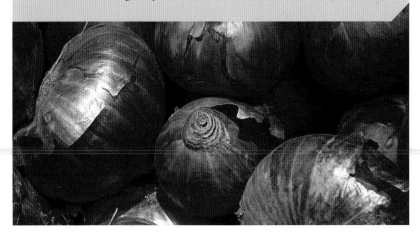

Leeks – are another of the allium family, delivering equal amounts of inulin.

Jerusalem Artichokes – contain a very powerful prebiotic called *fructo-oligo-saccharide* or FOS for short. This magical sugar goes way beyond the call of duty of most prebiotics. Rather than just being a food source for the good bacteria, it contributes to gut healing. When the gut bacteria feed upon FOS, they actually ferment it down, and convert it into a fatty acid called *butyric acid*. Butyric acid actually stimulates the regrowth of epithelial (inner lining skin) cells of the gut wall, leading to a stronger, healthier colon. This can be especially useful for anyone who has had problems with Candida to help heal the mess that it leaves behind.

Fennel and Rocket (Arugula) Salad with Mint Dressing

This is a beautiful, light, summery dish. It is packed full of crunch and vibrant, aromatic flavours.

1 fennel bulb
1 large handful of rocket (arugula) leaves
5–6 cherry tomatoes
5–6 slices of cucumber
1 large handful of mint leaves
4 tablespoons extra virgin olive oil
1 tablespoon apple cider vinegar

Finely shred the fennel in a large bowl. Add the rocket (arugula) leaves, tomatoes, and cucumber.

Dressing

Add the mint leaves, oil, and cider vinegar to a food processor, along with a pinch of crystal salt. Blend for 30 seconds.

Serve as a side salad to any of the dishes in this section, to further enhance the overall effect on digestive health.

MEDICINAL PROPERTIES

Fennel – is one of the most famous herbs for digestive complaints. It contains a whole cocktail of essential oils that give it its characteristic aniseed smell. These complex chemicals are powerful antispasmodics. This means that they help to relax the muscular walls of the gut. Many digestive complaints involve excessive or irregular episodes of the normal contraction of the gut wall. Diarrhoea and cramping gas feature these

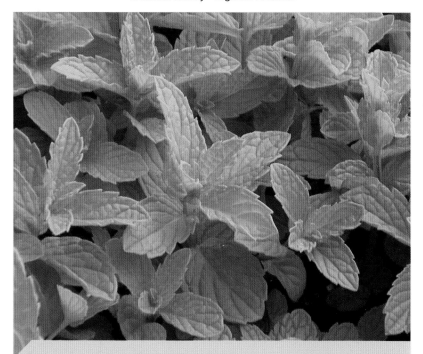

excessive powerful spasms. Antispasmodics help to relieve these symptoms very quickly and help to restore normal peristalsis.

Rocket (Arugula) – as many of you will know, is a very bitter-tasting vegetable indeed. This bitter taste is the key to its medicinal activity. Bitter foods such as rocket (arugula) can directly stimulate digestion. When the tastebuds in our tongue detect a bitter flavour, there is a natural reflex of two of the nerves that supply the tongue – the vagus and the hypoglossal nerves. These nerves also connect to the stomach and liver. When this reflex occurs, we naturally start to produce more digestive fluids in the stomach, and the gall bladder contracts harder, releasing more bile. This will help with the digestion and absorption of fats. This is also great if we may have been abusing our livers somewhat (i.e. after Christmas), as it can assist in the removal of waste from the liver. When the liver processes toxins ready for removal from the body, it alters them chemically, for easier removal. Those that it can make water-soluble will be removed via the kidneys and urinary system, and those that are chemically fat-soluble will be removed from the liver, via the bile, out of the bowels.

Mint – is a very rich source of an essential oil called *menthol*. This powerful oil, often used in cold and flu remedies, is also a powerful antispasmodic. It also helps to restore intestinal contractions to their normal rhythm much faster than any other natural ingredient.

Apple Cider Vinegar – is an old folk remedy for just about any condition you could possibly imagine. From digestive problems to arthritis, apple cider vinegar was believed to be the magic cure-all. While some of these claims may prove to be a little far-fetched, apple cider vinegar is certainly beneficial for digestive health. The vinegar is basically made from cider which has been allowed to ferment further to go from alcohol to vinegar. During this process, several beneficial acids are formed, including acetic, lactic, and malic acids. These acids work as natural prebiotic agents, encouraging the growth of good bacteria.

▶ Top Ingredients for the Digestive System

Artichokes – stimulate the liver to release bile, which helps carry away toxins.

Bay Leaves – help to relieve painful wind.

Beetroot – liver tonic, detoxifier, good for improving fat digestion.

Fennel – antispasmodic, helps to regulate contraction of the gut wall.

Garlic – helps to support growth of good bacteria.

Jerusalem Artichokes – greatly stimulate the growth of gut bacteria.

Mint – helps break down gas, and regulate contractions of the gut wall.

Rocket (Arugula) – stimulates bile flow, so helps improve fat digestion, and removal of toxins.

▶ General Dietary Tips for Digestive Health

▶ **Fill up on fibre.** I know there may be many of you who are dreading what's coming next; if so, relax. I'm not going to expect you to live on boxes of dry cereal and endless cracker breads that taste like jazzed up cardboard. The key to upping your fibre intake is simply to move towards a wholefood diet. This means that if you eat pasta, go for the brown wholemeal variety. Likewise with bread. Eat fresh fruit and vegetables, without cooking them half to death (choose steaming, stir frying, or eat them raw), and fill up on pulses such as lentils and beans.

So, why is fibre so important? Fibre basically helps to regulate digestive function in two ways. Firstly, unlike refined foods that just turn into a sticky paste, high-fibre foods provide some density to physically push material through the digestive tract. Secondly, fibre absorbs water, to create a stool that is larger and fluffier. This bulkier gut content starts to stretch the gut wall. Buried within the gut wall are thousands of stretch receptors. Once these receptors detect that the gut wall is stretching, they cause the muscle that lines the gut wall to contract, enhancing our normal peristalsis.

▶ **Drink plenty.** Sorry, I'm not referring to the Merlot here. I am referring to water, of course. As described above, high-fibre foods absorb water to become larger and bulkier, thus improving peristalsis. One rule here though, we need to be drinking enough of the clear stuff in the first place. Your body will always give priority to hydration of the brain and other organs, so if you aren't drinking enough, any water in the gut will be taken up into the body to properly hydrate the vital organs. This will make gut contents a lot harder, move through slower, and be more problematic to pass.

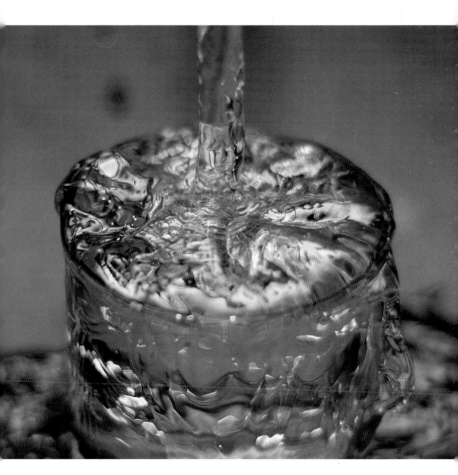

The Heart and Circulatory System

The circulatory system is literally our body's lifeline. Every tissue in our body requires a constant supply of oxygen and nutrients. Even seconds without such a supply would be life-threatening. This system comprises the heart, arteries, veins, and capillaries. There are, in fact, two circulatory systems in the body. The first is our main systemic circulation that travels throughout the length and breadth of our body. The second is the pulmonary circulation. This is a loop-like system. When the blood delivers its oxygen to tissues, the deoxygenated blood needs to return to the lungs, in order to receive a fresh load of oxygen from the air that we breathe. The heart is the most sophisticated pumping system in existence, never matched by any advances in technology. It beats 60–100 times per minute, 100,000 times a day, 30 million times per year, and 2.5 billion times in a 70-year lifetime. That's pretty impressive stuff!

Every single day, the equivalent of over 2,000 gallons of blood is pumped around the body. This staggering amount moves through over 60,000 miles of blood vessels, moving through every single tissue and structure throughout our body. Some are thick, wide arteries, some are blood vessels so thin and delicate, only a laboratory microscope can see them. This whole system is responsive to chemical messages that tell it how to perform in order to deliver more or less blood to different tissues, as their needs change.

Heart and circulatory disease is the biggest killer in the Western world – fact! In the UK alone, one in every four men, and one in every six women, will die from the condition, and over 300,000 people will have a heart attack this year!

There are two major risk factors to consider when looking after the long-term health of the heart:

Hypertension – refers to elevated blood pressure. The pressure within the blood vessels is constantly changing. The body needs to be able to alter the pressure within the circulatory system. This is to allow for higher or lower oxygen needs in different physiological circumstances. If a tissue needs oxygen at a faster rate, an increase in pressure within the blood vessels supplying that tissue will allow blood to fire in far quicker. The pressure changes in a blood vessel are controlled by rings and bands of muscle within the walls of the vessel that contract and relax, in order to change the internal size of the vessel, and therefore the vessel's volumes. Simple physics tells us that if we change the volume of the vessel without reducing its contents, the pressure within it will increase.

In the case of hypertension, the pressure within the blood vessels is high enough for long enough to increase the risk of "vascular injury". The elevated pressure in the blood vessel can lead to damage or rupture of the delicate inner lining of the vessel. When this happens, the lining will start to bleed, and, just like any other injury or scrape, a scab will form. Small cells in the blood, known as platelets, start to stick to the area of injury and produce a fibrous mesh to hold them in place, and literally plug up the hole. This scab that forms within the vessel is known as a thrombus. Due to the constant motion of blood moving through the vessel, this scab can easily be dislodged and can travel through the circulatory system. As the vessels spread out, they become narrower and narrower. Eventually, this scab will reach a vessel that is too narrow to accommodate it. When this happens, the thrombus will block the vessel and stop the blood flowing through it. This is when a heart attack or stroke arises. Learning how to lower blood pressure naturally is a powerful measure to introduce for the long-term health of the heart.

High cholesterol – in the human body is a hotly debated phenomenon. Many say that it is a stark indicator of heart disease risk, whereas others say that new evidence suggests that it has very little link with susceptibility to heart disease. Cholesterol is a vital substance in the body, not to mention one that is greatly misunderstood and feared. It is involved in manufacturing hormones, maintaining the outer walls of cells, and insulating nerve fibres. Cholesterol is formed in our liver from dietary fats.

Cholesterol in itself is not a harmful substance. What is important is the level of things called *lipoproteins* that affect the way in which cholesterol behaves in the body. Lipoproteins are essentially transporters that piggy-back cholesterol around the body. LDL, or low-density lipoprotein, carries cholesterol away from the liver through the bloodstream to the cells of the body that need it. If this lipoprotein is too high, it can lead to elevated levels of cholesterol in the blood, which can ultimately cause an unhealthy build-up of cholesterol in certain areas of the body, the most serious being within the vessel walls. HDL, or high-density lipoprotein, has the opposite effect. It carries cholesterol away from the body's tissues, via the circulatory system back to the liver, where it is broken down and removed from the body. This, in turn, helps to reduce the amount of cholesterol in general circulation, so lowers any chance of deposits forming within the vessel walls. It is in our best interest to encourage the elevation of HDL and the lowering of LDL. LDL can sometimes also be at risk of coming under attack by free radicals. These mischievous biological compounds attack other compounds and tissues to try to steal their oxygen. When this happens to LDL, it makes it highly likely that the LDL will be deposited into the blood vessel wall.

The main reason why the build-up of fatty deposits, or narrowing of the blood vessels, is an issue is simply that it affects the flexibility and integrity of the lining of the blood vessels. As we discussed earlier, the blood vessels can open and close, change diameter, with ease, in order to allow for changes in blood flow. If there are deposits within the vessel walls, their flexibility is reduced and the lining is impaired. Now, with this in mind, if the pressure within the vessel moves beyond a certain threshold point, because there is reduced flexibility and a weakening of the vessel walls, the likelihood of rupture or internal injury to the vessel wall is increased, making a heart attack or stroke more likely.

Recipes

Protection against heart disease is in many cases purely lifestyle-related. The foods that we eat can have a massive impact upon our likelihood of developing heart disease. There are many ingredients that can target different risk factors for heart disease. The following recipes are examples of the type of dishes that can easily and effectively be incorporated into your weekly or daily programme.

Celery, Carrot, and Ginger Juice

A quick, easy drink that can help to reduce blood pressure, and give a zingy vibrant start to your day.

2 sticks of celery
2 carrots
1 apple
2.5 cm (1 inch) piece of ginger

Simply run all the ingredients through a juicer – and that's it!

MEDICINAL PROPERTIES

Celery – is a fantastic source of many minerals and electrolytes, including magnesium. Magnesium helps to encourage the natural relaxation of the muscles in the blood vessel walls. It works side by side with calcium to regulate the contraction and relaxation of all muscles in the body. Calcium makes muscle fibres contract, whereas magnesium makes the fibres relax. Increasing dietary sources of magnesium can help to encourage this natural physiological occurrence.

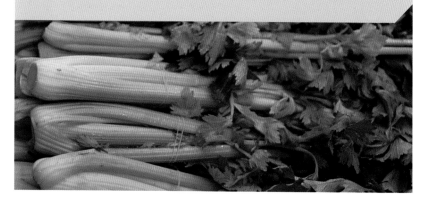

Celery also contains some fantastic chemicals, especially an interesting group called *coumarins*. These are part of the chemistry that gives celery its distinctive aroma, and are the same chemicals that give that wonderful smell when grass is being mown. Coumarins make celery act as a powerful diuretic. This means that it increases the level of urinary output. When urinary output increases, the distribution of fluids within the body changes, and the watery portion of our blood decreases. This means that the physical volume of the blood decreases. Then, simple physics kicks in – when the volume within a vessel decreases, the pressure within the vessel also decreases. This makes blood pressure go down for a while. This effect doesn't last all day, so celery should be a regular part of your diet for best results.

Ginger – is a great circulatory stimulant. It contains a powerful group of spicy compounds called *gingerols*, the compounds that give ginger its familiar spicy flavour and aroma. These compounds can cause a rapid and noticeable widening of the blood vessel walls. This is because they have an interaction with certain types of receptors within the inner lining of the vessel that causes the muscular walls of the vessel to relax suddenly. This has two distinct benefits – it can help to enhance circulation and also to lower blood pressure.

Carrots – contain a powerful chemical called *beta carotene* that is responsible for their bright orange colour. This compound is a powerful anti-inflammatory and has been shown to be incredibly protective to the cardiovascular system. It is believed that inflammation is at least partly responsible for the onset of injuries to the internal lining of blood vessels. Therefore, it is vitally important to ensure we have a good intake of anti-inflammatory foods such as carrots.

Edamame Bean and Chilli Dip

This gorgeous dip is mean, green, and ever so keen! I love it! It is really nice with raw veggie sticks, corn chips, rice cakes, or my favourite – on the end of my finger! It is packed with heart-healthy ingredients.

2 handfuls of fresh or frozen edamame (soy) beans
1 clove of garlic, finely chopped
1 fresh green chilli
3 tablespoons extra virgin olive oil
Celtic sea salt to taste
Handful of fresh coriander leaves (optional)

Another one of those joyously easy recipes – add all the ingredients, except the coriander leaves, to a blender or food processor, and blend into a smooth luxurious dip. Roughly chop the coriander leaves and add to the dip. Salt to taste, then get stuck in!

MEDICINAL PROPERTIES

Edamame Beans – are soybeans which have gained a reputation as a mild but effective cholesterol-reducing agent. A recent study in China has shown that the chemical compounds in soya, known as isoflavones, can cause the lowering of LDL cholesterol, and a concurrent raising of HDL cholesterol. It is also believed that it can inhibit the production of "new" LDL cholesterol. Edamame beans also contain chemicals called *phytosterols*. Phytosterols help to reduce the amount of cholesterol that is absorbed via the digestive system, thus helping to reduce total cholesterol.

Garlic – that old faithful! The strong-smelling sulphur-based essential oils in garlic have a longstanding reputation for encouraging the body to convert LDL cholesterol into HDL. There is also the presence of ajoene, a chemical that can reduce the activity of clotting factors. Clotting factors are chemicals that encourage the clotting and coagulation of the blood, so reducing their activity can offer protection against heart attacks and strokes.

Chilli – is one of those great all-rounders, with beneficial properties for virtually every single body system. Like ginger, chillies are a potent circulatory stimulant. The fiery-tasting chemical, capsaicin, which is found in the seeds and inner skin, stimulates the muscles in the blood vessel walls to relax. You may have eaten food with a lot of chilli in the past and experienced that sudden flushing and redness that can occur. This is the circulatory stimulating action of capsaicin, working its magic.

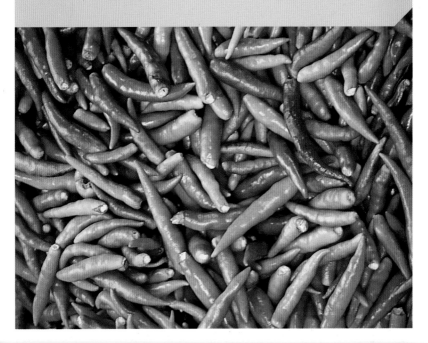

Shiitake and Sunflower Pâté

A gorgeous smooth, mushroomy pâté that is divine spread on crackers, toast, or as a dip for veggies. Its deep, earthy flavour keeps people coming back for more and more.

1 punnet of fresh shiitake mushrooms
3 tablespoons raw sunflower seeds
2 cloves of garlic
3 tablespoons extra virgin olive oil
Dash of soy sauce

This is the easiest dip in the world to make. Just throw it all into a food processor and blend into a smooth dip. That's it! No... really... that's actually IT. Season to taste. You can add more oil if you would prefer a slightly thinner dip.

MEDICINAL PROPERTIES

Garlic – among other things, garlic contains a powerful antioxidant that is believed to prevent LDL (bad) cholesterol from oxidizing. It is this process that causes cholesterol to clog up arteries, so anything we can do to stop this has got to be a winner. There are also sulphurous chemicals present that are believed to affect the production of this "bad cholesterol" transporter, thus leading to a greater presence of the "good" HDL.

Garlic also contains a potent compound called *ajoene*. This chemical has an interaction with a biochemical messenger called *platelet aggregation factor*. This compound tells the platelets in the blood to stick together and form a blood clot. The ajoene found in fresh garlic helps to lower heart attack risk in general, although we must note that this protective effect comes from prolonged use.

Shiitake Mushrooms – these amazing Asian treasures have long been known as a powerful stimulant to the immune system, and are commonly used in flu-fighting potions and soups, etc. However, many recent clinical trials in China and Japan have shown that shiitake may offer a protection against high cholesterol. This is due to the presence of a compound called *eritadenine*. Eritadenine appears to be able to encourage the conversion of the bad LDL cholesterol into the good HDL cholesterol, and also to give a general lowering of blood lipids (fats).

Sunflower Seeds – these gorgeous seeds are a fantastically rich source of a group of plant chemicals called *phytosterols*. These are the chemicals made famous by the myriad of cholesterol-lowering drinks, yogurts, spreads, etc, on the market. They essentially help to reduce the level of cholesterol taken up by the digestive tract. Cholesterol moves around our body in a bit of a loop system. It is made in the liver from specific dietary fats and then transported throughout the body via several mechanisms. One mechanism, in particular, involves cholesterol being released from the liver into the digestive tract, where it is reabsorbed into the general circulation. Phytosterols actually block this reabsorption, thus allowing the cholesterol in the gut to be removed from the body via the bowel. The cholesterol lowering activities of phytosterols have been very well documented in recent years, thus adding to their popularity.

Spicy Chickpeas

SERVES 1

I love this dish. It is a simple, easy, and incredibly tasty side dish that has many benefits for a healthy heart and cardiovascular system.

2 cloves of garlic, finely chopped
2.5 cm (1 inch) piece of ginger, peeled and finely chopped
1 fresh green chilli, chopped
1 can (400 g/14 oz) chickpeas, drained
½ teaspoon ground cumin
½ teaspoon ground coriander
½ teaspoon ground turmeric
½ teaspoon garam masala
½ teaspoon ground cinnamon

1. Heat about 2–3 tablespoons of olive oil or coconut oil in a pan on a high heat. Add the garlic, and allow it to turn brown in order to capture a smoky flavour.

2. At this point add a couple of pinches of sea salt or Himalayan crystal salt. Then, add the ginger and chilli, and allow to cook for a minute or two, until the ginger begins to get more fragrant.

3. Add the drained chickpeas, and mix thoroughly. Add all of the ground spices, apart from the cinnamon. Mix thoroughly again, and allow to simmer away for about 2 minutes. At this stage, take off the heat, and stir in the cinnamon.

MEDICINAL PROPERTIES

Chickpeas – contain a whole chemical cocktail that is beneficial to heart health, including saponins, lignans, and phytosterols. The most well understood of the bunch are the phytosterols. These are the same compounds that can be found in the myriad of cholesterol-lowering spreads and drinks. They help to lower cholesterol by actually binding to it, and carrying it out of the body via the bowel. They are also a rich source of magnesium, which can help to lower blood pressure and regulate heart rhythm.

Garlic – is the staple ingredient for a healthy heart. Just to re-emphasize, it is a powerful protective agent for reducing blood clots. The complex chemistry that gives it its pungent aroma is also a great regulator of cholesterol production, not to mention deliverer of a potent antiviral action.

Chilli – is a powerful vasodilator, which means that it can help to widen the blood vessels, increasing blood flow. It contains a chemical known as capsaicin, which causes a sudden and forceful relaxation of the blood vessel wall and consequently a notable drop in blood pressure.

Turmeric – is a well known anticoagulant (preventer of clotting), and is also a potent anti-inflammatory. The yellow pigment in turmeric helps to control inflammation, so can give significant protection against inflammatory damage of the inner lining of the blood vessels.

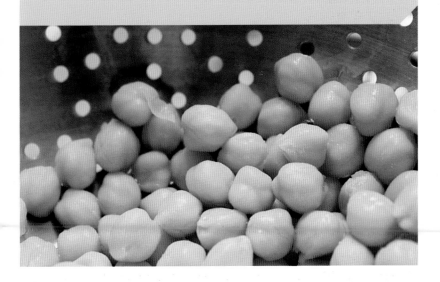

Spicy Lentil and Coconut Soup

SERVES 1

I love this dish. It's great as a winter warmer, and tastes like a tropical paradise!

2 tablespoons olive oil
2 cloves of garlic, finely chopped
1 red onion, finely chopped
1 spring onion, chopped
1 fresh green chilli, chopped
1 piece of fresh lemongrass, outer layers removed and finely chopped
100 g (3½ oz) red lentils
200 ml (7 fl oz/just over ¾ cup) coconut milk
Juice of half a lime

1. Heat the oil, garlic, onions, chilli, and lemongrass in a pan, and sauté for 5 minutes. Salt to taste using unrefined sea salt or Himalayan crystal salt.

2. Add the lentils, and pour in the coconut milk, along with 400 ml (14 fl oz/1⅔ cups) of water. Reduce the heat and let the soup simmer for 45 minutes, until the lentils are soft and mushy.

3. Remove from the heat, and squeeze in the juice from half a lime.

MEDICINAL PROPERTIES

Red Onions – contain a group of chemicals called *flavonoids* that are responsible for the deep red colour. These offer significant protection against excessive inflammation, which has been linked to the onset and progression of arterial disease. Onions also contain a chemical called *diallyl* *sulphide,* which has been shown to reduce clotting factors in the blood, thus offering protection against heart attacks and strokes.

Red Lentils – are very rich in both soluble and insoluble fibre. Both of these fibres are useful for carrying away cholesterol that is lurking in the digestive system, and removing it from the body via the bowel. Lentils are also a great source of magnesium that helps to relax the muscular walls of blood vessels and thereby naturally lowering blood pressure. Lentils also provide lashings of B vitamins, which help to maintain the health of the arteries and veins.

Garlic – is the superstar of many of the recipes in this book. It helps to reduce the blood's ability to clot, and encourages the production of the "good" HDL cholesterol, while reducing the levels of LDL.

Chilli – is a very powerful circulatory stimulant and a useful aid in lowering blood pressure. This is because of the powerful chemical, capsaicin, which forces the blood vessel walls to open, enhancing circulation and lowering blood pressure.

Lemongrass – is another powerful vasodilator that helps to widen the blood vessels by relaxing their muscular walls. This reduces the pressure in the vessels, and lessens the likelihood of injury to the internal lining of the vessels.

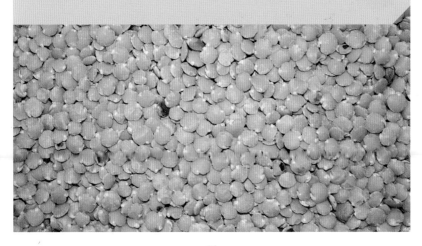

Red Ratatouille and Bulgar Wheat Stack

SERVES 4

This dish looks fabulous (see top dish on page 2), is light, and is packed with some exciting plant chemicals that are known to be beneficial in the reduction of LDL cholesterol.

2 handfuls of dry bulgar wheat
1 teaspoon vegetable stock powder
3 tablespoons olive oil
1 red onion, finely diced
2 cloves of garlic, finely chopped
10 vine-ripened cherry tomatoes, chopped
1 red pepper, deseeded and chopped

1. Place the dried bulgar wheat into a pan and cover with water. Add the vegetable stock powder and bring to the boil.

2. In another pan, add the olive oil, onion, and garlic. Add a pinch of salt and sauté until the garlic and onion are soft.

3. Add the chopped tomatoes and chopped red pepper, and cook until the pepper has softened and the tomatoes have broken down to become a thick sauce.

4. On a serving plate, place a layer of the tomato and pepper mixture into a cooking ring mould or deep round cookie cutter. Pack in tightly to around the half way mark. Then, place a layer of bulgar wheat on top, all the way to the top of the mould/cutter. Carefully remove the mould cutter to reveal a two-layer stack.

5. Serve with a good dense side salad.

MEDICINAL PROPERTIES

Onions – have a million and one medicinal applications, but have been shown in many clinical trials to be especially beneficial to the health of the heart and circulatory system. They contain a group of compounds called *sterols*. These are the same plant chemicals that are added to the well known spreads and drinks that are designed to lower cholesterol. Sterols help to reduce the uptake of cholesterol through the gut wall. This can be cholesterol from foods, or cholesterol that has been made in the liver and released via the gall bladder into the digestive tract. Onions also contain a group of sulphur-type compounds that can help to reduce clotting in the blood, so offer a protective role against heart attacks and strokes. Red onions, in particular, have another protective substance to throw into the mix. The purple pigment that gives them their distinctive colour comes from a group of pigment chemicals called *flavonoids*. These help to protect the inner lining of the blood vessels from damage.

Garlic – is again another food with a myriad of medicinal uses. It has very powerful antioxidant activities, and, as such, is believed to prevent the bad LDL cholesterol from oxidizing. This oxidizing (chemical damage) increases the likelihood of LDL being deposited into the blood vessel walls. Garlic also contains the same sulphur-based compounds as onions, but to a much greater extent, so offers powerful protection against excessive blood clot formation, plus it has ajoene present to further enhance this activity.

Red Peppers – also contain the vivid colour pigment chemicals called flavonoids, mentioned above. These compounds are responsible for the red colour of the peppers. They are powerful antioxidant agents that, according to the *American Journal of Clinical Nutrition*, play a significant role in the prevention of atherosclerosis. Flavonoids are also notable anti-inflammatory agents, so with the new information abound regarding the link between inflammation and heart disease, adding anti-inflammatory foods to your daily diet is an absolute must.

Apple Jacks

MAKES 6–10

Isn't it nice to have the occasional sweet treat? And why shouldn't we? We should be able to have our small moments of decadence, and still be doing our health some good. Lovely, light, sweet, delicious apple flapjacks. One bit just won't be enough with these. A sweet treat that's great for you – does life get much better?

**2 fresh apples
3 tablespoons dark agave nectar
5 tablespoons walnut oil
180 g (6½ oz) porridge oats
25 g (1 oz) chopped dates
2 teaspoons cinnamon**

1. Preheat the oven to 180°C/350°F/Gas mark 4.
2. Purée the apples in a food processor.
3. Add the agave and the walnut oil to a pan, and place on a medium heat. Allow the two to mix thoroughly.
4. Add the oats and chopped dates to the oil and agave nectar, and mix thoroughly until the oats are moist.
5. Stir in the apple purée and mix thoroughly.
6. Press the mixture into a greased baking tin and bake for around 25–30 minutes.
7. Sprinkle the cinnamon on top, cut into squares and devour.

MEDICINAL PROPERTIES

Oats – have so many great health-giving properties, from being a rich source of B vitamins, to stabilizing blood sugar levels. Oats are a great food. In the context of heart health, they contain a soluble fibre known as beta glucan. This compound is known to lower cholesterol levels by binding to

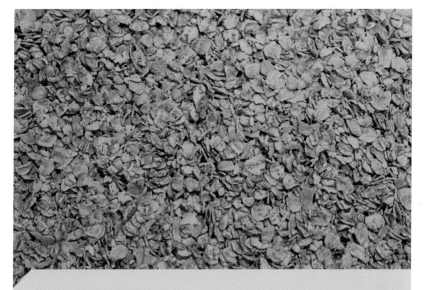

the bad LDL cholesterol, and then carrying it out of the body via the bowel. Beta glucan is also a great immune booster too, known to enhance white blood cell production.

Apples – have long been renowned to keep the doctor away. Apples contain a type of soluble fibre known as pectin. You may have come across pectin if you are a fan of making your own jams. It is used as a natural gelling agent. Pectin, just like beta glucan, binds to cholesterol and carries it out of the body via the bowel. The story doesn't end there, however. There is also a group of chemicals present in apples called *polyphenols*. These are also believed to lower LDL cholesterol, possibly by influencing the production of HDL over LDL. The final magic ingredient in apples is a substance called *ellagic acid*. This helps to break down excessive cholesterol in the liver, and also protects cells from damage, which has got to be good.

Chocolate Orange Truffle Torte

No, your eyes haven't deceived you, and, yes, you are still reading the same book! I created this dish simply to prove that healthy food can also be a decadent, delicious, and delightful affair. Why should we feel like we are missing out on something, just because we choose to eat healthily? This recipe is just as delicious as your gourmet restaurant equivalent, and I have even given it to people without telling them what it was made from, and they thought I'd finally cracked and given in to some naughty treats – they nearly fell off their chairs when I told them what went into it!

Base:

200 g (7 oz) raw mixed nuts
30 g (1 oz) melted raw cacao butter
2 tablespoons agave nectar

Filling:

2 soft, ripe hass avocados
1 large orange
2 tablespoons agave nectar
50 g (2 oz) raw cashew nuts
3 heaped tablespoons raw cacao powder
30 g (1 oz) melted raw cacao butter

Base

Add the mixed nuts to a blender. Blend into a coarse powder. Using a glass bowl nestling in a pan of water placed upon a medium heat (think back to the days of melting chocolate for Rice Krispie cakes), melt the cacao butter. Add this to the blended nuts, along with the agave nectar, and mix thoroughly. Press this mixture into a flan tin, or cheesecake tin, as if you were making a cheesecake base. Also allow the crust to go up the sides, so it makes something similar to a flan case. Place the lined tin into the freezer to allow the cacao butter to set rapidly.

Filling

Scoop out the avocado flesh into a food processor. Grate the rind of the orange into the food processor, then half the orange, and squeeze its juice in as well. Then, add the agave nectar, cashew nuts, and the raw cacao powder, and blend until a smooth, rich, chocolate pudding-like texture is reached. At this stage, it's back to the stove to melt the second batch of cacao butter. Once melted, add this butter to the other mixed ingredients, and process on a lower setting until the butter is evenly mixed. Remove the tin from the freezer, and scoop the chocolatey filling into the semi-set base. Spread out evenly, and then place in the refrigerator for 4 hours.

The base will set to a biscuity texture, and the filling will reach a texture like firm chocolate mousse. One taste of this and you will feel like all of your birthdays have come at once!

MEDICINAL PROPERTIES

Nuts – are packed to the hilt with many amazing compounds and nutrients. They are a very rich source of the mineral selenium. This vital nutrient is used by the body to make its own natural anti-inflammatory enzymes, mainly SOD (Superoxide dismutase). This enzyme is also believed to be a part of the body's own natural protection mechanisms against damage to arterial walls. Many nuts have also been shown to have significant LDL-cholesterol-lowering properties. This may be due to the fact that many nuts are high in the compound oleic acid. This is the same chemical that is found in olive oil, and is responsible for olive oil's cardio-protective properties.

Avocados – again, these are a very rich source of oleic acid, which has notable effects upon lowering cholesterol. Avocados are also a very rich source of vitamin E, which can help to protect against excessive blood clotting, and also helps to reduce chemical damage to fats that are circulating in our blood. Chemical damage to these fats can cause injury to blood vessel walls and increase the likelihood of clot formation.

Oranges – contain a group of compounds called *bioflavonoids*. These are found in the rind and pith of the orange, and are known to protect the inner lining of blood vessels from damage. They do this by strengthening the microscopic mesh that holds all the cells together within the lining. This mesh is found in every solid body tissue and is known as the "extracellular matrix".

Cacao (Raw Chocolate) – is awash with over 1,500 active chemicals that can have an amazing impact upon our health. In the context of heart health, though, raw chocolate has two major benefits. Firstly, it is an incredibly dense source of the vital mineral magnesium. Magnesium is involved in regulating heart rhythm. It is also used, alongside calcium, in maintaining and regulating muscular relaxation and contraction. Calcium causes muscle fibres to contract, whereas magnesium causes them to relax. The walls of the blood vessels are made up of many layers of muscle. Increasing our intake of magnesium can play a role in maintaining a healthy blood pressure. The second major benefit of cacao is the incredibly high antioxidant content. Even though chocolate appears brown, it is in fact a very deep purple colour. This is an incredibly dense concentration of plant pigments that deliver powerful antioxidant benefits. This is useful, because it helps to protect blood vessels from damage, and reduce the oxidization of cholesterol.

▶ Top Ingredients for Heart Health

Apples – carry away cholesterol, encourage cholesterol breakdown in the liver.
Celery – diuretic, helps to lower blood pressure.
Chilli – vasodilator, lowers blood pressure.
Garlic – converts LDL to HDL, reduces risk of clotting, antioxidant.
Ginger – vasodilator, helps lower blood pressure, reduces risk of blood clot.
Onions – protect vessels from damage, reduce clotting.
Chickpeas (and all pulses) – high in sterols, help to remove LDL cholesterol from the body.

▶ General Dietary Tips for Heart Health

While there is an abundance of individual ingredients that can have a powerful influence upon specific factors of heart health, there are also some changes in diet and lifestyle that can have a drastic affect on the health of the heart and circulatory system. The good news is that they are easy to adopt. Heart disease is thankfully something that is incredibly responsive to changes in diet and lifestyle. Even the smallest changes can have a massive impact upon our risk of heart disease, not to mention a drastic improvement in any damage or issues that may already be present.

▶ **Reduce saturated fat intake.** The first dietary change to make is reducing your saturated fat intake. This means cutting back on foods such as red meat, hard cheeses, milk, and cream. All dietary fats influence the manufacture of certain products in our body. This could be the production of communication molecules called *prostaglandins* that regulate the inflammatory response and pain signalling. They also determine which types of cholesterol/lipoprotein complexes are formed. Saturated fat encourages the production of LDL, the bad cholesterol carrier, which, in the long term, can lead to fatty deposits on the artery walls. By changing the type of fats we consume, we can alter the levels of the good and bad cholesterol carriers.

However, there is actually a bit of a dichotomy to this rule. I would advise anyone to give up vegetable spreads tomorrow! No, actually, do it now! There have been huge amounts of mass marketing to persuade us to give up butter, in favour of margarine, in order to "protect us" against the dreaded dangers of saturated fat. Granted, all I said above is most certainly true. However, there is an abundance of new evidence that suggests that the margarine spreads are drastically worse for us than saturated fat could ever be. This is because they contain hydrogenated fats. Vegetable oils are naturally liquid at room temperature. To get them to look and behave the same way as butter, manufacturers have to bubble hydrogen gas through the oil. This essentially changes the chemical structure of the fat, and turns it into a semi-solid spread. This change in chemical structure creates something that the body has an almost impossible task to recognize and deal with once we consume it. New data coming into the spotlight in recent years suggests that the consumption of such spreads is actually worse than butter. What do I recommend? I'd use butter every time. The body knows what it is, and how to deal with it. Just be sensible how much you use.

▶ **Plant-focused diet.** The second, and probably single most important, tip for a heart-healthy diet is to drastically increase your intake of fruit and vegetables, with the emphasis being on the veggies. Fresh plant foods are abundant in vitamins, minerals and antioxidants, which all are pivotal to the general health of our body. Antioxidants, in particular, can help to reduce damage to tissues such as blood vessel walls.

However, the nutrients in fresh plant foods are just the very beginning of the story. Fresh plant foods contain a whole cocktail of active chemicals that aren't nutrients, but are very powerful medicinal compounds. These foods are also naturally low in fat, and fill you up for longer.

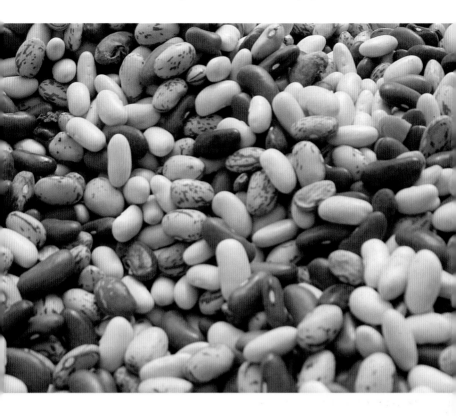

▶ **Increase high-fibre foods.** The third diet tip is to up your intake of high-fibre foods, like wholegrains and pulses. These foods contain high levels of both soluble and insoluble fibre, which can help to bind to cholesterol and carry it out of the body. These foods also make you feel fuller faster, so can be a great weight-loss tool too.

The Immune System

Like an aggressive army of complex, highly organized specialist units, our immune system is our attack and defence mechanism, and the keeper of the peace within the challenging and often lurid landscape of our internal environment. Every single day, we are completely bombarded with a whole host of bacteria, viruses, fungi, toxins, and parasites that would all love the opportunity to live and thrive in our organs and tissues. There are hundreds of ways that these little miscreants can find their way into our body. Thankfully, there are just as many ways for our immune system to keep them out. However, our immune system's work does not end there. This intricate system can also detect things such as our own cells turning cancerous, and can destroy them before they get a chance to cause too much mischief. This mechanism can sometimes be reduced by certain environmental influences, which is when a tumour is given the opportunity to flourish.

The immune system never stops working and, most of the time, we will be completely unaware that anything is going on inside us at all. The only time we really become aware of it is when our immune system is caught "off guard" and we get an infection such as a cold or an infected cut, or when our immune system's response causes us a physical symptom, such as the itch from a mosquito bite or the symptoms of allergy such as hay fever.

The system as a whole is made up of an immaculately regulated network of cells, tissues, and organs that work in unison to provide a multifaceted defence against all manner of biological and physiological challenges.

The white blood cells

White blood cells, technically called *leukocytes*, are probably the most well known part of our immune system, and are responsible for most of the immunological activity in our body. They circulate through the bloodstream, through our organs, and also through the lymphatic system (the filtration system that carries waste away from our tissues).

Leukocytes are divided into two distinct types. These are *phagocytes* and *lymphocytes*.

Phagocytes are essentially a type of white blood cell that can identify and destroy a pathogen that can potentially cause a problem. A phagocyte stretches itself out until it is able to completely swallow up an invader. Once it engulfs it, the phagocyte pulls the invader inside itself. When inside, the phagocyte releases a whole host of chemicals to attack and break down the invader until it has been completely destroyed. The remains of the pathogenic invader are then "spat out" and safely removed from the body.

Lymphocytes make up the rest of the white blood cell population. There are two main types of lymphocyte: B lymphocytes and T

A leukocyte (white blood cell) known as a lymphocyte, magnified 1125X.

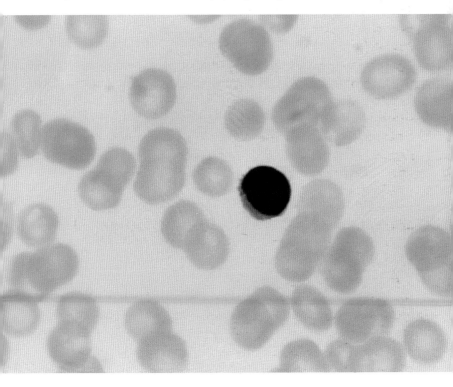

lymphocytes. The B lymphocytes can be likened to army intelligence. They actually seek out specific invaders and rally the troops. When they identify a specific invader, they begin to make "antibodies" for this invader. The antibodies made by B lymphocytes are then used to direct the activity of the immune system's response to this particular invader. T lymphocytes get involved in this part of the process by either producing chemical signals that recruit other cells and get them involved in the fight, or by releasing clouds of highly poisonous granules that can actually destroy cells that have become infected by the invader. During this whole process, B and T lymphocytes leave a lasting memory of the battle they waged when faced with that specific invader, in the form of things called *memory cells*, that store the specific antibodies to that particular invader. For the rest of our lives, these cells will "remember" this particular bug and, any time it tries to attack, our immune system will know how to handle it before it even gets a look in. It is on this basis that our childhood immunizations work.

The lymphatic system

The lymphatic system is the filtration system for all of our body's tissues. It consists of a huge network of vessels, very similar to those in the circulatory system. The lymphatic system also features filtration stations called *nodes* and areas of lymphatic tissue that help to keep an eye on what is happening in the body.

In all of our tissues, between each and every cell, in all the minute spaces, is a liquid that bathes the tissue called *interstitial fluid*. This fluid is part of the transport medium that allows nutrients to enter cells and for waste to be removed from the cells. Once a tissue cell excretes its waste, it enters the interstitial fluid. The interstitial fluid flows away from the tissues and into the lymphatic vessels. Once this fluid enters the vessels, it is then known as "lymph". The lymph is carried along the vessels by contraction of the vessel walls that occur when we move our bodies (another reason why exercise is so important). This fluid and all the waste products it contains eventually finds its way out of our bodies, via the kidneys and urinary system.

The story doesn't end there. The lymphatic system also plays a major role in immunity. Remember the B and T lymphocytes we talked about earlier? Well, the lymphatic system is their primary hang out (*lymph* – lymphocyte), and one of the routes that they use to get around the body. The lymphatic system also transports a group of cells called *antigen presenting cells*, which help to identify certain invaders in our body. The biggest assistance to the immune system, however, is the filtration devices present in the lymphatic system, called *lymph nodes*. These nodes, often mistakenly called *glands*, are the things in your neck, armpits, and groin, that swell up when you are ill. When the doctor feels your neck and says, "Your glands are up", that means there is inflammation within the lymph nodes. Essentially, the lymph nodes are a very fine filter that can trap all manner of pathogens, from bacteria to viruses, and unwanted biological detritus, such as toxins and cancerous cells that may be circulating around the body. Once these unwanted items become trapped in the lymph nodes, the cells of the immune system are called to the scene to get rid of whatever the filter has trapped. When all this punishment is taking place, inflammation occurs within the node and, hey presto, your "glands" are up!

Other means of defence

While the mechanisms described above make up the bulk of the body's defence system, there are other means employed by the body to protect itself.

The population of friendly bacteria in the gut is one of our body's first lines of defence against pathogens that find their way in through our mouth. Most simple bacteria will be destroyed by the highly volatile and acidic environment of the stomach. Some, however, are able to get through. When these come into contact with the bacterial population of our intestinal system, a battle often ensues, as friendly bacteria assist in the destruction of these invaders.

The skin is another unlikely part of our immune system. It creates a very tough physical barrier to the outside world that very few pathogens can penetrate. The only time bugs can get through the skin is when there is already an opening such as a cut or graze.

Therapeutic management of the immune system

Stimulating white blood cells

White blood cells, like any other body tissue, are drastically influenced by any changes in the internal environment of the body. There are compounds present in foods that can slow our white blood cells right down, almost putting them "to sleep". On the same note, there are compounds in foods that can drastically stimulate the activity of white cells. When stimulated in this way, white cells actually seem able to move to the site of infection much faster, and also respond to pathogens and infected tissues in a far more aggressive manner. There are also naturally occurring compounds that can stimulate the tissues that manufacture white blood cells to work even harder, increasing the actual production of these cells.

Managing inflammation

Whenever we get an infection, cut ourselves, or have any type of damage or injury in our body, inflammation will always become active at one stage or another. Inflammation in and of itself is far from a negative thing, it is actually a vital part of the healing process. However, it also rapidly runs away with itself and can cause a great deal of discomfort. Much of the symptom patterns that we experience during infections are caused by the inflammatory process. Whether it is a blocked up nose, a tight chest, painful diarrhoea, inflammation will always be playing its part.

While we don't want to switch off inflammation permanently, learning tricks to manage its severity can play a huge role in making us feel that little bit better.

Garlic Honey

This is one of the easiest recipes in the world. It is great to make in the midst of a cold, or something that you can make in advance, and store in your medicine cabinet. This recipe is particularly effective in cases of sore throats and throat infections such as tonsillitis.

Fresh garlic cloves
UMF 15 manuka honey

This recipe doesn't call for specific measurements, just a simple ratio.

1. Chop the garlic very finely, as small as you can get it. Then, simply cover with double the amount, by volume, of the manuka honey, and the same amount again of water.

2. Mix all three ingredients well, and leave for 2–3 days onwards. The mixture will get stronger and more potent, the longer it is left to infuse.

    Dosage: take 1–2 teaspoons of this mixture every 2 hours during cold or flu infection.

MEDICINAL PROPERTIES

Manuka Honey – has gathered legendary status in recent years when it comes to dealing with colds, flu, and infections. In some cases it is given almost panacea-like qualities that, if accurate, would make us immortal. While there has been a lot of hype surrounding manuka honey, there are certainly some positive attributes. It is a honey produced by bees that constantly visit the flowers of the manuka bush.

Like all honeys, manuka is high in a chemical called hydrogen peroxide, which is a highly reactive substance. When the honey coats the back of the throat, the hydrogen peroxide content will start to decompose bacteria quite rapidly and render it harmless. Please note, however, that this effect is only observed on surfaces that the honey touches directly.

The thing that sets manuka honey apart from any other is the presence of a widely studied compound called *UMF*, or *Unique Manuka Factor*. This compound, thought to be derived from the manuka bush itself, has been shown to be a powerful antibacterial agent. This effect is observed both locally and systemically, meaning that not only does it deliver its effects to surfaces that it comes into immediate contact with, but also throughout the body as a whole.

Garlic – is probably the global king of herbs for any kind of infection. Garlic contains a very potent group of sulphur-based essential oils – the bit responsible for the lingering smell. These oils do not get broken down by the body, and can only be removed via one waste removal route – the breath. As these essential oils move through the respiratory tract, they are very effective at destroying viruses and bacteria.

These oils are made stronger and are more highly activated when garlic is crushed or finely chopped.

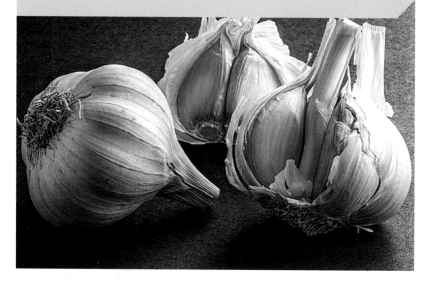

Goji and Pumpkin Seed Energy Bombs

They provide a simple and easy snack, high in nutrients and energy, that can be eaten at any time of the day. They are especially useful if you are suffering from the sniffles, as they are packed with immune-boosting chemicals and nutrients.

1 heaped tablespoon coconut oil
3 handfuls of pumpkin seeds
3 handfuls of goji berries

The method for making these tasty treats will probably remind you of making cornflake cakes as a child.

1. Quarter fill a saucepan with water and place a heatproof glass bowl on top to create a bain marie (remember melting the chocolate for those cakes?). Add the coconut oil to the bowl.

2. Meanwhile, add the pumpkin seeds and goji berries to a food processor, and process at a medium speed to get a coarsely ground texture.

3. Begin to melt the coconut oil in the bain marie. Once melted, add to the processed goji berries and pumpkin seeds, and mix thoroughly. This will give a sticky but firm mixture. Roll into bite-sized balls, place onto a plate, and refrigerate until firm.

MEDICINAL PROPERTIES

Goji Berries – have been in the world media in recent years, with some rather astounding and notably far-fetched claims being made about them. They have been viewed as the ultimate superfood. While much of the

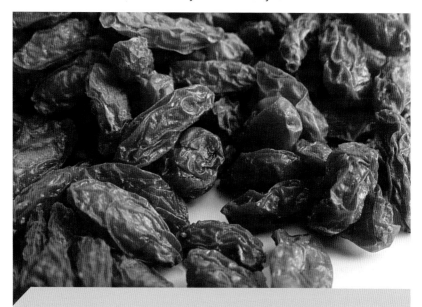

media attention can realistically be considered hype, goji berries do certainly have some interesting effects upon the immune system. Like many medicinal plants and mushrooms, they contain a group of special sugars called *polysaccharides*. These sugars are discussed in greater detail in the following soup recipe. However, they are known to be a very powerful stimulator of the immune system. They do this by causing an increase in the production of white blood cells.

The second thing about goji berries, and the thing that I find most interesting, is their high levels of the trace element *germanium*. Germanium is one of the hardest trace elements to find in our modern diet and is one of vital importance when it comes to the health of the immune system. Germanium is an important nutrient in the regulation of a group of cells called *CD4 cells*. These cells can be viewed as almost like the conductor of an orchestra. They essentially tell all other cells of the immune system what to do, when, and how, and play a pivotal role in the organization of almost every immune response. It is the CD4 cell that is affected by HIV infection, and a decline in these cells is what causes the immune system's demise in this awful disease.

Pumpkin Seeds – are definitely one of my favourite nibbles to have around the house. They are very high in another important trace mineral: zinc! Zinc has been widely researched in recent years, especially in the context of immunity. One of the key roles that this wonderful mineral plays is the regulation of the functioning of individual white blood cells. It does this by ensuring correct functioning of their individual DNA – the internal code that programs every function of every cell in every tissue. A healthy, fully functioning DNA means a healthy fully functioning white blood cell, able to deliver its best performance when faced with an invader.

Pumpkin seeds are also a very rich source of the chemical cucurbitin, which is a powerful antiviral and anti-parasitic agent. This makes it very useful for things such as food poisoning, where the infective agent has found its way into the body via the digestive tract. Pumpkin seeds have a longstanding history as a traditional remedy for such infections.

Flu-Fighting Soup

SERVES 3–4

This soup is an absolute powerhouse when it comes to dealing with the symptoms of cold and flu. It is a one-pot wonder. Easy and speedy to make.

1 red onion
2 green chillies
4 cloves of garlic
5 cm (2 inch) piece of ginger
1 small butternut squash
1 punnet of shiitake mushrooms
Vegetable stock

1. Finely chop the onion, chillies, garlic, and ginger. Add to a pan with a little olive oil, and a pinch of crystal salt. Sauté on a mid to high heat until the onion softens.
2. Dice the butternut squash, discarding the seeds. Slice the shiitake mushrooms. Add these two ingredients to the onion, garlic, chilli, and ginger. Stir well, then add enough vegetable stock to cover all the ingredients. Simmer well, until the squash is soft.
3. At this stage, add the soup to a blender, and blend into a vivid orange, spicy soup.

MEDICINAL PROPERTIES

Butternut Squash – is a very rich source of the antioxidant compound beta carotene. This is the plant form of vitamin A and the chemical responsible for the vivid yellow flesh of this delectable squash. Beta carotene is a subtle but effective anti-inflammatory, which can help reduce the severity of generic cold and flu symptoms.

Butternut squash also contains a compound called *cucurbitin*. This is a very strong antiviral and anti-parasitic chemical. It is found in very high concentrations in pumpkin seeds, but also in the membranous, stringy flesh that is found in butternut squash (in the area that the seeds are removed from).

Shiitake Mushrooms – have been used as a tonic for the immune system for centuries. They have been highly revered in traditional medicinal systems of the Orient. You may well be wondering what is so special about a simple mushroom. The truth is that certain types of mushroom can deliver a stronger influence to the immune system than any other substance, natural or manmade.

Medicinal mushrooms, such as shiitake and maitake, contain a group of very chemically complex sugars called *polysaccharides*. Almost 40 years of clinical study in Japan, USA, and China, has revealed that these sugars are the magic bullets that make medicinal mushrooms such powerful immune boosters. It was once believed that these sugars were absorbed by the body and then caused the immune system to behave a certain way. However, it is now becoming clear that these sugars exit the body via the bowel completely untouched, yet the effect is still being observed. If you recall the description of the lymphatic system above, you will remember that there are areas of lymphatic tissue around the body performing certain functions. In the walls of our gut, there are patches of lymphatic tissue called *Peyer's patches*. These can be likened to surveillance stations in the gut, keeping an eye on what is going on. These stations are staffed by a team of cells called *dendritic cells* that constantly monitor what is going on in the digestive tract, as it is a convenient way for bugs and pathogens to enter the body. Dendritic cells are powerless to deal with any type of invader or troublemaker themselves, rather, they are able to effectively identify the type of problem, then quickly and conveniently radio through to the right emergency service that can deal with the problem. It is believed that when the polysaccharides found in shiitake mushroom move past these patches of tissue in the digestive tract, they cause the dendritic cells to become excited and release chemical messengers that rush through the whole body and cause a sudden and drastic increase in the production

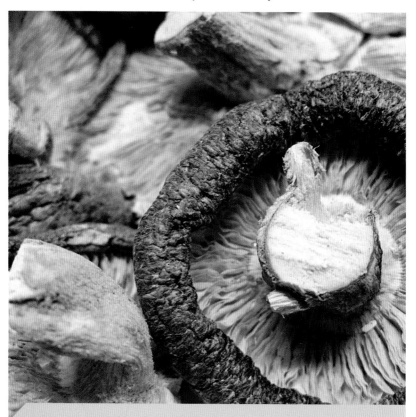

of white blood cells. This is because the polysaccharides have a similar chemical shape to sugars expressed by some common types of bacteria. In essence, by eating these mushrooms we dupe the body into thinking that it is under a more serious bacterial attack. Obviously, as we aren't, this response gives us more of an abundance of white blood cells that are then able to move towards the site of infection from colds, flu, etc, and deal with the problem far quicker.

Consumption of these mushrooms on a regular basis is a great way to enhance our daily defences, even when we are not sick.

Garlic – is the mother of all natural antivirals. The strong smelly oils help to kill viruses and bacteria in the upper digestive tract.

Ginger – is another one of those ingredients that we naturally associate with cough and cold medicines. Ginger has a wide and complex chemistry. Part of this is a group of compounds called *gingerols*. These essential oils, that give ginger its strong zingy aroma and spicy flavour, are well known as strong anti-inflammatories. Similar to a class of drugs known as COX-2 Inhibitors, the oils found in ginger help to interrupt the inflammatory process. When inflammation becomes active, a series of chemical reactions takes place, with the end result being active inflammation. Gingerols simply get in the way of this chain reaction and prevent it from becoming fully active, thus naturally lowering inflammation.

During a cold, we can experience an uncomfortable bunged up feeling: a blocked nose and congested sinuses. Many of us think that we are bunged up with mucous (there is obviously some present), but most of that feeling actually comes from inflammation of the mucous membranes that line the nose and sinuses. The anti-inflammatory action of ginger helps to reduce the bunged up sensation.

The second benefit of ginger is that it stimulates circulation, by relaxing the blood vessel walls and widening the vessel. Enhancing circulation in this manner helps to increase the rate at which white blood vessels move around the body on their way to the site of infection. It also increases the rate of delivery of fresh oxygen and nutrients, and the removal of waste products from all tissues, including those that are infected.

Chilli – has been used medicinally by almost every conceivable traditional medicinal system on planet earth. Apart from its powerful stimulatory activity, and painkilling properties, chilli can rapidly thin out mucous, making it far easier to remove from the body. This is especially useful when we are so bunged up that we can't even blow our nose. I'm sure many of you have experienced the classic runny nose after eating a strong chilli. Consuming these as much as possible during an infection can really help to clear things up rapidly.

▶ Top Foods for a Healthy Immune System

Chillies – help to thin mucous.
Garlic – one of the most renowned antivirals on earth.
Ginger – reduces inflammation of mucous membranes.
Goji Berries – contain immune-boosting polysaccharides that increase white blood cell numbers.
Manuka Honey – powerful antibacterial properties.
Pumpkin Seeds – rich sources of zinc. Antiviral properties.
Shiitake Mushrooms – powerful immune stimulators. Boost white blood cell numbers.

▶ Dietary Tips for a Healthy Immune System

▶ **Avoid refined sugar.** Simple, refined sugars, such as the white sugar that you may put in your tea, white breads, and white pasta, are terrible for our health on so many levels. Sugar and refined carbohydrates are renowned for greatly reducing our immunity. Studies have shown that even an intake of around 35 grams of sugar (about the amount you would find in a can of fizzy drink) is enough to cause a fifty per cent reduction in the ability of phagocytes (a specific type of white blood cell) to be able to engulf and destroy bacteria. Sugar is also known to slow down the rate at which white blood cells migrate to the site of infection, and is also believed to slow down the production of white blood cells in the thymus gland. If you need to use sweeteners, go for things such as raw agave nectar, yacon syrup, or a good quality honey. Swap white bread, rice, and pasta, for the wholegrain varieties.

▶ **Eat the rainbow.** Brightly coloured fruits and vegetables are often the magic bullets for all round health. Each vivid colour represents different spectrums of phytochemicals and antioxidants. Many of these brightly coloured compounds help to protect tissues from damage,

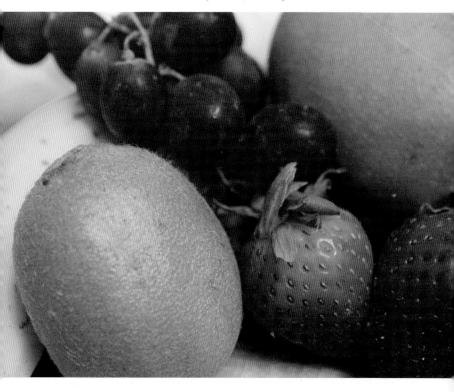

reduce inflammation, and give the immune system a helping hand by enhancing the overall health of the tissues in general.

▶ **Stay hydrated.** Staying properly hydrated is important for many reasons. In the context of immunity, being properly hydrated will help in the removal of waste products from the body. This will, of course, take a certain amount of burden away from tissues, so will help to leave them healthier and less open to infection.

The Joints

The joints – where two bones meet and the connective tissues within them – are the most extensively used structures in our bodies. Joints allow flexibility of various parts of the body. They give us movement and help us in creative expression. We can run, and jump, and dance, and take gentle walks in the countryside.

The movement of our joints is given by the movement muscles which pull on tendons that are attached to our bones. Cartilage covers the ends of bones to ensure there is a smooth cushion for the two bony surfaces when they move. Most fully movable joints in the body are what are known as "synovial" joints. This means that they are surrounded by a fluid-filled sack that allows for a more full range of movement and articulation. Between the cartilage of two bones which form a joint there is a small amount of thick fluid called *synovial fluid*. This fluid "lubricates" the joint and allows smooth movement between the bones. The synovial fluid is made by the synovium. This is the tissue that surrounds the joint. The outer part of the synovium is called *the capsule*. This is tough, gives the joint stability, and stops the bones from moving "out of joint". Surrounding ligaments and muscles also help to give support and stability to joints.

Now, throughout our lifetimes, the joints and connective tissue within them can take an awful lot of abuse and be subject to a lot of wear and tear. This, naturally, depends a great deal on the type of activities we engage in. Athletes, for example, are at far greater risk of experiencing joint issues in later life than those who engage in moderate exercise. Of course, doing no activity at all can be equally as detrimental, since exercise has a bearing upon bone density, plus a sedentary lifestyle is more likely to cause someone to hold many extra pounds, which can in itself put increased burden upon the joints.

The degree of physical wear and tear is not the only lifestyle factor that can affect the health of our joints. Our internal environment has a huge part to play. This is where dietary influences can have a massive impact, and certain foods can provide a powerful, safe, and delicious intervention.

Therapeutic Management of Joint Problems

In virtually every circumstance, joint problems centre around two major factors: inflammation and over activity of the immune system (often referred to as "auto-immune"). These must be taken into consideration when creating a medicinal menu for joint problems. We also need to consider other ways in which we can help the body to manage symptoms, such as increasing and supporting the activity of the lymphatic system and the kidneys.

Management of Inflammation

In every known joint malady, there is an inflammatory involvement to one degree or another. This inflammation may be caused by a whole host of different reasons. Whatever the cause, inflammation is the primary factor for pain and joint immobility. The body produces many of its own chemical agents that are used to "switch on" an inflammatory response, as well as chemical agents that inhibit inflammation. These can be substances called *prostaglandins*, other substances called *cytokines*, and also a third group of compounds called *free radicals*.

The most significant and easy to manage of these chemical agents are fatty substances called prostaglandins. Prostaglandins are chemicals manufactured in our bodies from fats. They are involved, among other things, in activating or regulating the inflammatory response in our bodies. Many pharmaceutical anti-inflammatory drugs work by directly influencing prostaglandins or the chemicals in the body that manufacture them. There are three main types of prostaglandin: series 1, series 2, and series 3. Series 1 and 3 are very powerful anti-inflammatory agents that can quickly and effectively reduce inflammation and pain. Series 2, on the other hand, actually instigate the inflammatory response and its associated pain.

The good news, however, is that we can manipulate which of these our body makes the most of. The raw ingredients for the manufacture of prostaglandins in the body are fats. A diet high in saturated fat – the type found in many meats, dairy produce, etc – will cause the body to manufacture a great deal more of the series 2 variety which, as we know, only really serve to promote inflammation and pain.

Conversely, a diet high in poly and mono unsaturated fats from food sources such as seeds, oily fish, olive oil, etc, will encourage the body to produce the series 1 and 3 prostaglandins that manage and minimize the inflammatory process. Our body will take the fats we consume in our daily diet and feed them through a series of chemical reactions. Depending upon the type of fat we consume, and its unique chemical structure, a specific inflammatory mediator will arise. Aside from manipulating the raw materials that the body uses to make prostaglandins, there are foods that we can eat which contain powerful chemicals that actually block some of the chemical processes involved in prostaglandin manufacture. Isn't nature amazing?

As mentioned above, there are also a group of chemicals called free radicals that also cause localized inflammation. Now, free radicals may sound like some sort of guerrilla military group, but they are, in fact, highly reactive oxygen molecules that rely on other oxygen-containing chemicals in the body to stabilize them. This can create all sorts of havoc. Free radicals have been associated with accelerated ageing, cancer, and excessive inflammatory states. The good news is that there are a very powerful group of chemicals abundant in nature that can help to keep these biological troublemakers under control. It is most likely that you will have heard of these substances before, as they have been all over the media in recent years, and have become somewhat of a fashionable buzz word. They are of course "antioxidants". Antioxidants help to diffuse the anger of free radicals, our biological miscreants, by simply giving them what they want – the electron that makes their oxygen stable.

The easiest way to ensure that we consume enough antioxidants is to focus upon brightly coloured fruits and vegetables. The deep colours, like the red in peppers, or the purple in beetroot, all represent different antioxidants, so a colourful plant-based diet is definitely the way to go for optimal antioxidant intake.

Control of immune response
Joint problems, such as osteoarthritis, arise due to normal wear and tear of cartilage within the joints. However, there is a specific type of

arthritis that is a completely different animal. That is rheumatoid arthritis. This is an auto-immune condition, which means that, for whatever reason, the body's own immune system has developed antibodies against its own tissues. In this case it is the cartilage and connective tissues within the joint capsule. Now, the immune system has two main ways of responding. These are non-specific and antibody-mediated responses. Non-specific immunity refers to when the immune system recognizes anything as being "foreign" or non-self, or recognizes one of our own cells that has become diseased or infected. Antibody-mediated reactions, on the other hand, involve the body indentifying a bacteria or invader of some kind, and creating antibodies to it that act like a memory. So, if a specific antigen is experienced again, the immune system knows how to deal with it. This is all well and good until it goes awry and produces antibodies to our own tissue.

Thankfully, there are some unlikely foodstuffs that can dramatically reduce the impact of antibody-mediated immune responses. One food, in particular, has been the subject of thousands upon thousands of studies for its effect upon the immune system. This is the shiitake mushroom!

Diuresis (increasing urinary output)
As previously explained, most movable joints in our body have a sack of fluid that envelopes the two ends of bone. The fluid, known as synovial fluid, is present to lubricate and nourish the tissues within the synovial capsule. This fluid receives nutrients and expels waste produce, via the lymphatic system (sometimes called *the body's second circulatory system*). Normal day to day metabolic functions within the joint capsule can leave behind waste products and gunk that the immune system can react to. This causes tissue damage and localized inflammation, thus causing pain and reduced joint movement and, if left unattended, damage of the tissues within the joint.

It is vital, therefore, that we enable these waste products to be cleared from the joint and the body as rapidly as possible. This is achieved by increasing the rate at which waste material travels out of the joint capsule, into the lymphatic system, on to the kidneys, and out of the body through the urine. Certain herbs, foods, and ingredients can stimulate the activity of the kidneys and lymphatic system. This action is known as diuresis. Stimulating the kidneys' expulsion of fluid from the body in essence speeds up the removal of all fluid bound waste products from the body, as general movement of fluid in the body speeds up somewhat. Ingredients such as parsley, celery, dandelion, and fennel all have very strong diuretic capabilities.

Pineapple, Celery, and Ginger Smoothie

This recipe is a fantastic all rounder. It is of relevance to every type of joint malady imaginable and so easy to make. I find it a great breakfast option for a lot of my clients, and one that they themselves make, day in, day out, purely because it gets quite addictive.

½ large fresh pineapple
2 fresh celery stalks
2.5 cm (1 inch) piece of fresh ginger root

1. Prepare the pineapple by cutting off each end. Then, slice off the skin in a downward direction. This minimizes waste. Remove "eyes" from the flesh of the pineapple, and then cut half of the flesh into manageable chunks.
2. Chop the celery stalks into small pieces.
3. Peel the ginger and chop finely.
4. Place all the ingredients into a blender, along with a tiny amount of water, and blend into a smooth fragrant drink.

MEDICINAL PROPERTIES

Pineapple – contains a very powerful enzyme called *bromelain*. This has well documented anti-inflammatory properties. It controls inflammation by interfering with several chemical messengers that are directly involved in the production of series 2 prostaglandins (the inflammation instigating chemicals discussed above). Bromelain also helps to control the role that the immune system plays in inflammatory damage. It seems to be able to reduce the number of neutrophils that migrate to the affected area. Neutrophils are a type of aggressive white blood cell that becomes highly active during inflammatory attacks. Bromelain is found in the highest concentrations in the slightly tougher inner core of the pineapple. Many people discard this piece, but make sure you don't if you want to pack the greatest anti-inflammatory punch.

Celery – is probably the most seemingly innocuous food on the planet. I bet most of you wouldn't credit it with much in the way of medicinal benefit. In reality, however, celery is a powerhouse of complex chemicals. It contains a compound called *3-n-butylphthalide* (*3nB* for short). This substance is a very potent anti-inflammatory and a notable painkiller. OK, granted, its effects aren't exactly comparable to strong pharmaceuticals like ibuprofen, but celery is a perfect example of the type of food that can be added to your daily regime that will give cumulative benefits to support and enhance that of your medication. Celery also contains a wonderful group of chemicals called *coumarins*. These are the same chemicals that fill the air with that gorgeous distinctive smell when a lawn has just been mown. The coumarins in celery are known to help remove metabolic waste products that can accumulate within the synovial capsule of the joint. Once removed, these by-products enter the lymphatic system where they are sent to the kidneys for removal via the urine.

Ginger – is, without doubt, the crown king of anti-inflammatory ingredients. Ginger contains a powerful group of chemicals that give it its characteristic zingy flavour and aroma, including two chemicals called *zingerone* and *shogaol*. These are both powerful anti-inflammatory agents. They work in a similar way to a class of pharmaceutical drugs known as COX-2 inhibitors. These drugs work, again, by interfering with the production of pro-inflammatory prostaglandins. Ginger also acts as a very powerful circulatory stimulant, so can be of great use in easing discomfort in cold, stiff joints.

Garlicky Hemp Seed Dip

This fast, easy recipe is a divine alternative to foods like hummus. I love it with things like corn chips, celery sticks, and flax seed crackers. It is packed to the hilt with compounds that regulate inflammatory processes and also substances that help to support the structures within the joints.

150 g (5 oz) raw shelled hemp seeds
3 tablespoons extra virgin olive oil
1 clove of garlic, finely chopped
Pinch of Celtic sea salt

Add all the ingredients to a food processor, and blend into a deliciously smooth dip. You may add extra olive oil to achieve your preferred texture. Salt to taste, and process for another 10 seconds. And that's it.

MEDICINAL PROPERTIES

Hemp Seeds – are one of the few foods in nature that provide a perfect balance of essential fatty acids. We have all heard about fatty acids like omega 3, 6, and 9 in recent years, and the multiple benefits that they supply. However, in order to get these benefits, we need to consume them in the right ratios. We need to consume twice the amount of omega 3 than omega 6, especially if we want to achieve the anti-inflammatory effects, described above, that these fats can deliver. Hemp provides huge amounts of fatty acids, and the good news is that it provides them in the perfect ratio for nature to get to work and manufacture those anti inflammatory compounds.

Hemp is also a great source of zinc and selenium. These two vital minerals help the body to create its own natural antioxidant compound called *glutathione peroxidase*, which can help to buffer inflammation too.

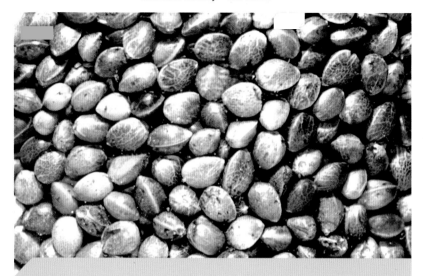

Garlic – has so many medicinal properties, they could easily fill a whole book. When it comes to joint health, garlic contains huge amounts of sulphur. This vital compound makes up to 75 per cent of all connective tissues, such as those found within the joint structure as ligaments and tendons. Getting a good dietary source of sulphur can offer great nutritional support to these tissues to ensure they remain strong and supple.

Rainbow Salad

SERVES 1

This is great for any inflammatory condition and is a fantastic health-boosting side salad for anyone. I have added it in the joint health section for the simple reason that it is absolutely packed to bursting point with inflammation-zapping antioxidants.

2 slices of red cabbage
1 carrot
½ red pepper
1 handful of baby spinach
Small handful of parsley

For the dressing
1 clove of garlic
1 teaspoon honey
2 teaspoons dark soy sauce
2 tablespoons extra virgin olive oil

1. Prepare the salad by shredding the cabbage, grating the carrot, finely chopping the pepper, and adding to the whole baby spinach leaves and parsley.
2. Prepare the dressing in a small bowl. Finely chop the garlic, add a pinch of salt and all the other wet ingredients. Mix well, and pour over the salad. Toss the salad well, and serve.

MEDICINAL PROPERTIES

Red Cabbage – has a very strong antioxidant activity. This is due to the vivid purple pigments that give it its distinctive colour. They are a group of chemicals called *anthocyanins*. These are similar chemicals to those found in red wine. Anthocyanins can help to reduce inflammation in any tissues by supplying an antioxidant buffer.

Carrots – are also rich sources of a strong antioxidant known as beta carotene. This substance is responsible for carrots' vivid orange colour. This is also the same chemical that gives the colour pigment to yellow peppers. There is just a far lower concentration present. Beta carotene is the plant form of vitamin A. Our bodies can convert it into vitamin A as and when it needs it. Aside from this, beta carotene is also a strong and easy to obtain antioxidant.

Parsley – has notable diuretic properties. It contains a strong essential oil (which contributes to its strong smell), that actually acts as a very mild and harmless irritant to the kidneys' filtration systems. This gentle irritation increases urinary output, which will help the body to remove waste products from the joints far more quickly.

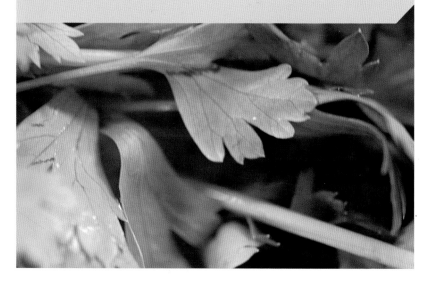

Dandelion Salad

SERVES 1

This is a slightly unusual but thoroughly satisfying salad that is fabulous for the health of the joints and a great cleanser on all levels. This is due to its strong diuretic action from the dandelion, celeriac, and the celery. It is possible to buy dandelion leaves pre washed and packed from some supermarkets, but it is most likely that you will need to collect them by hand from the wild, which is great fun and also brings a whole new relationship between you and your food. Just make sure you pick healthy-looking, deep-green ones, preferably far away from a busy road.

1 stick of celery, diagonally chopped
½ carrot, grated
2 tablespoons grated celeriac
3 tablespoons alfalfa sprouts
1 large handful of dandelion leaves, thoroughly washed
1 teaspoon pumpkin seeds
1 teaspoon sunflower seeds

Dressing
1 tablespoon pesto
2 tablespoons extra virgin olive oil

1. Blend the vegetables together, and mix with the dandelion leaves.
2. Mix the olive oil and pesto together thoroughly and pour over the salad. Sprinkle the seeds over the salad and mix again.

MEDICINAL PROPERTIES

Dandelion Leaves – are just fabulous. These nutritionally dense leaves are an extremely effective diuretic agent. We have already established that diuretic substances are useful in removing the metabolic waste that can be left lying around following inflammatory activity. This action from dandelion has been documented for centuries, and dandelion leaf is often called upon

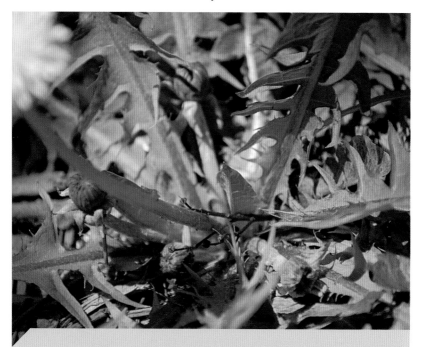

by herbalists for problems such as fluid retention and as a strong detoxifier. However, it is still unknown exactly how this effect takes place. Many people believe that it is due to the mineral content of these lush leaves and how those minerals affect the rate at which the kidneys allow fluids to move out of the body.

Celery – tends to feature in a lot of my recipes, simply because it has a very complex chemistry, with broad-reaching physical properties. There is a chemical present in celery called *3-n-butylphthalide* (*3nB*). This substance has been used as a significant painkiller. Clinical trials have shown that this has a particularly beneficial effect in rheumatic and muscular pain. It is also believed that this compound can help to remove metabolic waste, formed by the inflammatory response, left behind in the joint capsule. This waste can sometimes trigger further inflammation, so its removal is favourable. This second effect is further enhanced by the presence of a group of chemicals called *coumarins*. These aromatic chemicals also work as a diuretic.

Carrots – are very rich in the antioxidant nutrient beta carotene. This nutrient will work as an anti-inflammatory agent. Some inflammatory responses are driven by powerful free radicals (biological bullies described previously). Antioxidant nutrients will put a stop to these devilish agents, as well as protecting the body from the damage that free radicals can do to tissues systemically.

Celeriac – this is the root of the celery plant and contains the same constituents as the aerial (above ground) parts, but in higher concentrations. The addition of this tasty aromatic root to the salad will further enhance the diuretic and pain-relieving properties that have been discussed for celery.

Pumpkin and Sunflower Seeds – these delicious seeds are a wonderful source of minerals, including the vitally important selenium. They also contain omega 3 and omega 6 essential fatty acids that are involved in moderating the inflammatory process by manipulating the production of those oh so important prostaglandins we have discussed several times in this section. The selenium found in pumpkin and sunflower seeds is an antioxidant and an anti-inflammatory compound.

Anti-Rheumatoid Risotto

SERVES 4–6

As the name of this dish suggests, this particular recipe is designed to help manage the painful symptoms of rheumatoid arthritis. Rheumatoid arthritis is believed to be an "auto-immune disease". The immune system normally makes antibodies (chemical messengers that help the immune system identify an invader that it has successfully dealt with before) to attack bacteria, viruses, and other foreign invaders. Once these antibodies are created, the immune system can then remember the invader and what type of biological attack successfully destroyed it. In auto-immune conditions, the immune system makes antibodies against tissues of the body, and subsequently mounts an almost continuous attack upon those tissues. It is not clear why this happens. Some people seem to have a tendency to develop auto-immune diseases. In such people, something might trigger the immune system to attack the body's own tissues. The "trigger" is not known, although some people believe that this could be anything from exposure to some kind of environmental influence, viral or bacterial infection, food sensitivity, or compromised gut function. However, as there are so many possible instigating factors, it is often best to support the way in which the body reacts to such conditions, rather than trying to isolate the single aggravating agent. In people with RA, antibodies are formed against the synovium (the tissue that surrounds each joint and lines non-cartilagenous surfaces). This causes inflammation in and around affected joints. Over time, the inflammation can cause damage to the joint, the cartilage, and parts of the bone near to the joint.

This delicious recipe contains some wonderful ingredients that are major players in the management of rheumatoid arthritis. These ingredients are anti-inflammatory, diuretic, and immunomodulating. These are the three main actions that herbalists would have in the forefront of their minds when developing a prescription for a rheumatic patient. Thankfully there are foodstuffs that also have these actions. Such recipes can support the medication given to you by either your herbalist or your doctor, and are perfectly safe in combination. And the recipe is delicious!

Vegetable bouillon
1 red onion
2 cloves of garlic
6 sun-dried tomatoes
1 stick of celery
Extra virgin olive oil
250 g (9 oz) Arborio risotto rice
8–9 dried shiitake mushrooms
Dash of white wine (the rest can be
your treat for working so hard in the kitchen)
Handful of fresh spinach leaves

1. Make up 1 litre of stock using the vegetable bouillon – I'd advise about 1 level tablespoon to 1 litre (2 US pints) of water.
2. Finely chop the red onion, garlic, sun-dried tomatoes, and the celery, plus a little salt. Sauté these in a large pan in a little of the olive oil until the onion is soft and becoming transparent.
3. Next, add the risotto rice to the pan and stir the onion mixture and rice together. Add to this just enough stock to almost cover the rice. Allow this to simmer constantly.
4. As the stock gets absorbed, keep topping it up until you are left with about 300 ml (10 fl oz) of stock.
5. At this point add the shiitake mushrooms. The reason that these are added in so late is to protect their active chemicals which can be damaged if exposed to extremes of temperature for too long.
6. Continue to cook in the same way – adding stock as the rice absorbs more and more. When all the stock has gone in, add the dash of white wine (maybe 80 ml/3 fl oz). Then allow the whole mix to cook down until the texture is close to a thick oatmeal texture, and the rice is soft. At this point add the spinach as it will wilt in seconds.
7. To finish, add a tablespoon of extra virgin olive oil to the mix and beat the mix until a creamy texture is reached.

MEDICINAL PROPERTIES

Red Onions – These contain strong anti-inflammatory flavonoid chemicals called *anthocyanins*. Inflammation is the key factor responsible for the pain and destruction within the joint in rheumatoid arthritis. Even though over activity of the immune system is the trigger, inflammation is that final factor that causes the greatest destruction within the joint.

Celery – as we have discussed in detail, is a very effective diuretic agent, and natural painkiller that has proved effective in two clinical trials so far, particularly in the treatment of rheumatic and muscular pains when taken internally.

Shiitake Mushrooms – These delicious fungal treats are almost miraculous when it comes to the effect they have on the immune system. In rheumatoid arthritis, the body's immune system develops antibodies to the synovial tissue within the joint, and certain cells within the immune system start attacking this tissue, causing inflammation and destruction. Now, the immune system has two very specific ways of operating. The first is antibody-mediated – where the immune system will recognize a certain

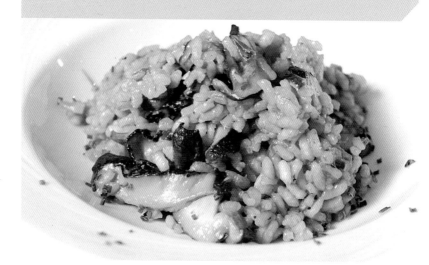

invader from past experience and mount a specific attack on it. It is this that is responsible for rheumatoid arthritis and other auto-immune conditions. The second is called *non-specific*. This means that the cells associated with it are able to tell if something is self (part of the body) or non-self (an invader or foreign substance). Shiitake mushrooms drastically stimulate the activity of the non-specific branch of the immune system. The good news here is that these two branches of the immune system are mutually inhibitory, meaning that they cannot both work at the same time. One counteracts the other. So, if the non-specific branch is stimulated, the antibody-mediated is suppressed!

Extra Virgin Olive Oil – that staple of Mediterranean cuisine, contains high levels of good fats which help the body to manufacture its own anti-inflammatory substances – the series 1 and 3 prostaglandins discussed earlier on page 89. These anti-inflammatory compounds are produced following correct metabolism of the right kinds of fat, and help to counteract the inflammatory responses that cause the pain, discomfort, and degradation within the joints in arthritic conditions. Regular consumption of this oil and other sources of good fats can play a huge role in the management of many inflammatory conditions, not just limited to those within the joints.

Anti-Inflammatory Curry

SERVES 4

This recipe is an anti-inflammatory powerhouse. It is suitable for any inflammatory condition, as it contains a powerful cocktail of ingredients known to tone down certain elements of the body's natural inflammatory responses. I have found that this dish seems to be of particular benefit to sufferers of osteoarthritis. Osteoarthritis, also referred to as degenerative arthritis, is the type of arthritis that occurs from ongoing wear and tear of the joint, and is more commonly (but not exclusively) associated with ageing. It arises from a wearing down of the cartilage that covers the two bone ends within the joints, and also a "drying out" of the synovial fluid, which provides joint lubrication. The resulting state is one where the unprotected surfaces of the bone then rub together in a coarse fashion, triggering inflammation, pain, and discomfort. While natural medicine provides us with some powerful remedies such as glucosamine that can offer massive relief from OA, foods and dietary changes can also provide relief from inflammatory attacks. This dish is a perfect example of this.

1 tablespoon olive oil
2 red onions, thinly sliced
2 large cloves of garlic, finely chopped
1 teaspoon freshly grated ginger
2 green chillies, thinly sliced
1 teaspoon ground coriander
1 teaspoon ground cumin
1 teaspoon black mustard seeds
1 heaped teaspoon turmeric
800 g (1¾ lb) sweet potato, diced with skins left on
375 ml (13 fl oz) vegetable stock
150 g (5 oz) spinach, coarsely chopped
Large handful of fresh coriander leaves, coarsely torn
1 tablespoon toasted flaked almonds

1. Heat the oil in a large saucepan and cook the onion, garlic, ginger, and chilli.
2. When the onion has softened, add all the spices and heat until they are becoming fragrant.
3. Add the sweet potato and stock and simmer for about 15–20 minutes until the sweet potato is soft. At this point add the spinach.
4. Once the spinach has wilted, the curry is ready to serve with coriander leaves, topped with flaked almonds. It is best served with brown rice to increase its nutritional profile further.

MEDICINAL PROPERTIES

Sweet Potatoes – are a great source of several anti-inflammatory compounds, some of which contribute to its wonderful orange-coloured flesh. The first of these is beta carotene. This is the same antioxidant chemical found in carrots, and most orange-coloured fruits and vegetables. This precursor to vitamin A is a strong antioxidant nutrient. This nutrient helps to combat the effect of these reactive molecules. The other compounds that work in a similar way are the flavonoids. Flavonoids are also strong colour pigments in the plant kingdom that give a colour spectrum ranging from deep reds, to oranges, to yellows. These too are potent anti-inflammatories and antioxidants.

There are also some unique proteins present within sweet potatoes. These are storage proteins that are held within the root as a source of nutrition for the plant to use as it grows. These particular proteins have potent antioxidant activity many times stronger than the carotenoids present, making this vegetable a significant anti-inflammatory ingredient.

Turmeric – has been used in traditional herbal practices for centuries. It is again a powerful anti-inflammatory agent. This is thanks to the chemical group known as curcuminoids. These substances make up turmeric's yellow

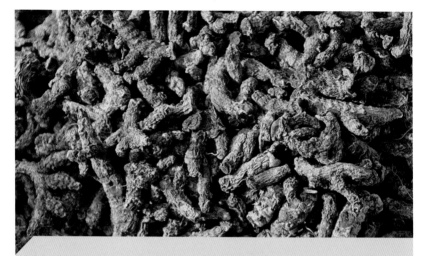

pigment (which stains your white shirt after a night at the curry house). The anti-inflammatory activity of these compounds has, in clinical trials, been shown to be comparable to such powerful drugs as hydrocortisone, phenylbutazone, indomethacin, and Nurofen. The anti-inflammatory activity of these compounds is due to their ability to inhibit the activity of a group of enzymes in the body that are responsible for certain stages of metabolism of dietary fats. Remember from the discussions above – fats are the precursors for the key substances prostaglandins. These are the compounds that can either cause inflammation and pain, or suppress it. The enzymes blocked by the curcuminoids are the ones that allow for the formation of the pro-inflammatory series-2 prostaglandins.

Ginger – is another well known ingredient that has been used in traditional medicine, the world over, throughout history. It is most commonly used in the treatment of nausea, and for improving circulation. However, in recent years it has emerged that ginger can have a very beneficial effect upon patients suffering with both osteo and rheumatoid arthritis. Patients have described a notable reduction in pain, and improved motility of the joint. The key component here is a group of chemicals known as gingerols. These compounds are again anti-inflammatory, but work in a different way from the other ingredients discussed so far.

In the introduction to this section, it was revealed that the immune system was also responsible for some degree of the inflammatory activity that arises in conditions such as arthritis and bursitis. The gingerols found in ginger actually interfere with the production of chemical messengers produced by the immune system, known as cytokines. These chemicals can signal all manner of events in the body. In this case, the types of cytokines that encourage inflammation are rendered inactive by the gingerols in ginger.

These few recipes hopefully give you some inspiration to create your own delicious and powerful recipes. Get in the kitchen and get creative, and make use of the most powerful medicinal ingredients for joint health.

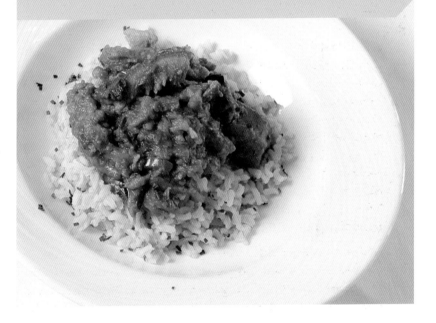

▶ Top Ingredients for Joint Health

Celery – painkiller, diuretic, anti-inflammatory.
Chilli – natural painkiller, circulatory stimulant.
Garlic – anti-inflammatory, source of dietary sulphur.
Ginger – anti-inflammatory, painkiller, circulatory stimulants.
Pineapple – anti-inflammatory.
Shiitake Mushroom – immunomodulator.
Sweet Potato – anti-inflammatory, immunomodulator.
Turmeric – anti-inflammatory, painkiller.

▶ General Dietary Tips for Joint Health

While there are some very powerful ingredients that can directly influence joint health, there are also general diet and lifestyle changes that you can make to further support the overall health of the joints. These changes are easy and can bring rapid results.

▶ **Reduce animal protein intake.** Don't worry, I'm not on some kind of crusade to turn the world onto any specific diet. There is, however, a vast amount of scientific data that shows a correlation between high consumption of animal protein and increased severity of inflammatory conditions. This is usually because animal proteins tend to be high in certain types of fats. If you recall our discussion of prostaglandins – the fat-derived inflammatory regulators – you will remember that some of them are anti-inflammatory, whereas some of them actually encourage and enhance the inflammatory response. Which ones the body creates is very much determined by the dietary fats we feed into the body. Animal fats are the type that the body uses to create the series 2 prostaglandins that worsen inflammatory conditions.

▶ **Reduce refined carbohydrates.** Refined carbs, such as white sugar, white bread, white pasta, white rice, etc, can play absolute havoc in the body. All other negative influences aside, refined carbohydrates can negatively affect the immune system, and can cause our white blood cells to behave rather erratically. It is believed that this can exacerbate some of the inflammatory processes instigated by certain white blood cells. Refined carbohydrates also cause fluctuations in hormones such as insulin, the knock on effect being an increased production in those nasty pro-inflammatory prostaglandins.

The Nervous System

The nervous system has to be one of the single most complex systems in the body. Its primary function is to coordinate and regulate activities in the body, and communicate signals and messages between different parts of the body. It is made up of the brain, spinal cord, and all the nerves that branch off this and supply all of the body's tissues. As such, the nervous system is divided into two distinct parts: the central nervous system (CNS) and the peripheral nervous system (PNS).

The CNS refers to the brain and spinal cord. It can be viewed as being the central computer, where all incoming information is processed, decisions are made, and commands are derived from. The central nervous system regulates every involuntary action in the body, such as breathing, blinking, etc. The brain attaches to the spinal cord, which then branches out many times, dividing off into the peripheral nervous system, in order to give nervous supply to all tissues and areas of the body. The spinal cord is, in essence, a thick collected bundle of nerves, giving a complete connection of the brain and body.

The peripheral nervous system is the branch of the nervous system that extends beyond the spinal cord and supplies all of our peripheral tissues. These are the nerves that tell the brain what is going on in the rest of the body and what is happening in our immediate environment.

Therapeutic management of nervous system disorders

Regulating nerve structure

Our nerve cells are made mostly of a very dense layer of fat. This fatty layer, called the *myelin sheath*, is vital in the normal communication between nerve cells. You may well know that nerve cells carry information in the form of an electrical signal. This electrical impulse moves along the nerve cell at lightning speed to carry messages and impulses from one part of the body to the other. To cut the travelling time of the electrical signal along the nerve cell, nature has created a wonderful method of conducting this signal. There are thick capsules of myelin sheath (fatty outer layer of the nerve cell, specially designed for carrying the electrical impulse), with small spaces between them.

These spaces are known as the "Nodes of Ranvier". When the electrical impulse is generated by the nerve cell, it jumps across these spaces (nodes), in order to cover a greater distance and a greater speed, thus ensuring that the communication between nerves takes place fast enough to keep every action and reaction running smoothly.

With the above in mind, we can see how important the structure of a nerve cell is in relation to its function. The fatty myelin sheath is pivotal to the nerve cell working properly. During normal day to day metabolic activity, the myelin sheath is constantly being broken down and rebuilt. Problems begin to arise, however, when the body's ability to rebuild the myelin sheath is surpassed by the natural breakdown that occurs. This can cause the nerves to have an impaired myelin sheath, which leads to problems with nerve cell communication. This can, thankfully, be addressed by supplying the body with the right types of fats. When we consume the right types of fat (such as the well known omega 3), we are actually taking in a very good source of the structural material that the body uses to lay down fresh myelin sheath. When we metabolize and break down omega 3, we produce two end products. These are EPA and DHA (eicosapentaenoic acid and docosahexaenoic acid). EPA is greatly involved in the regulation of inflammatory activity in the body. DHA, on the other hand, is a material used to maintain the structure of all cells in the body – especially myelin sheath in nerve cells.

Regulation of neurotransmitter production

As we have seen above, communication within the nervous system is, mostly, an electrical process, with impulses travelling along a nerve cell, jumping along the Nodes of Ranvier. However, nerve cells do not actually touch one another. There is a gap in between each one. The electrical signal that travels along the nerve cannot actually jump the gap between nerve cells. Therefore, once the electrical signal has travelled along the nerve, it has to come to a stop at the nerve endings, but one nerve still has to communicate with the next, in order to carry a signal or command along the whole nervous system, to or from the brain. In order to carry the signal across the gap between nerve cells (otherwise known as the synapse), the nerve cells have a bank of different chemical messengers stored up in their ends. These chemical messengers are called *neurotransmitters*. When the electrical signal gets to the end of one nerve cell, a cloud of these chemical messengers is released by one cell, and their message is received by the next nerve cell in sequence. This chemical message is then relayed, again, as an electrical impulse, which travels along the nerve cell to the next, and so the sequence continues. There are several types of neurotransmitter stored in nerve cells. The type of nervous signal being sent will determine which type of neurotransmitter is released.

There are certain foods, nutrients and phytochemicals that can actually influence either the production of these neurotransmitters in the body, or influence the way in which they are released or absorbed by nerve cells.

Cardamom and Banana Porridge

SERVES 1

This dish is absolutely beautiful. It tastes like a sweet, tropical paradise. You will feel like you are having breakfast in the Maldives. Not only is it warming and satisfying, it also has a wonderful impact upon the nervous system.

2 handfuls of porridge oats
300 ml (10 fl oz) rice milk
2 teaspoons powdered cardamom
1 banana, chopped

1. Add the oats, rice milk, and cardamom to a pan. Simmer, until a thick porridge is produced.
2. Transfer to a serving bowl, and chop the banana into the porridge.

MEDICINAL PROPERTIES

Oats – have been used in traditional Western herbal medicine for centuries. They have traditionally been used as a remedy for nervous exhaustion, anxiety, and prolonged stress. They have always been known as what herbalists call a "nutritive nervine". Oats have a very calming and centring effect on the nervous system that can be easily felt. The mystery is, however, what substance in the oats is doing this and how. They contain quite a complex chemistry, consisting of saponins, and alkaloids that all may have an influence on the nervous system to some degree.

Cardamom – has traditionally been used as a digestive remedy in Ayurveda – the traditional medical system of India. However, in recent years, it has come to light that the powerful fragrant essential oils responsible for the

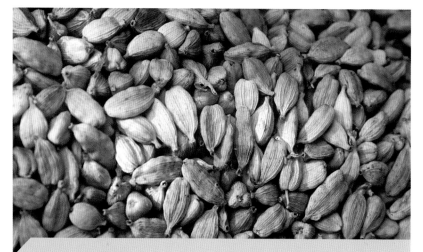

beautiful aromatic flavour of cardamom can actually influence the brain and nervous system. They do this by increasing levels of the neurotransmitter serotonin. This neurotransmitter, among other things, gives us that "feel good factor", and is the target chemical for many drug therapies for issues such as anxiety and depression. Cardamom influences serotonin by interacting with receptors in the digestive tract that causes a reflex action throughout the whole nervous system. The end result is an increase in the release of serotonin throughout the nervous system.

Bananas – are a very rich source of the mineral potassium. This is one of the most important minerals in regulating nerve function. It is involved in generating the electrical impulse that travels along the nerve cell. It does this by moving backward and forwards across the nerve cell membrane, carrying a current with it. Increasing our intake of potassium-rich foods, such as bananas, can notably improve overall nerve function.

Lavender and Rose Chocolate

SERVES 1

This recipe is absolutely divine. It's not very often that a health-related book actually encourages the consumption of chocolate, but this is definitely one of those rare exceptions to the rule.

This bar takes the already powerful mood-enhancing properties of chocolate to the next dimension.

1 large bar (about 100 g/4 oz) of 70% cocoa dark chocolate
1 teaspoon lavender flowers
5 drops of lavender essential oil
10 drops of rose essential oil

Remember the days, as a child, making cornflake cakes? Well, you are about to revisit them.

1. Break up the chocolate bar into small pieces, and place in a heat-proof glass bowl. Place the bowl in a pan of gently simmering water in order to create a bain marie. Allow the chocolate to melt.

2. At this point, add the lavender flowers and the two essential oils. Mix well, and then transfer to the moulds of your choice. You could make a single bar, or small bite-size pieces. I tend to use an ice-cube mould, so that I have little bite-size pieces to nibble on when I feel like a fix.

MEDICINAL PROPERTIES

Chocolate – is not the dastardly terrible food that people make out that it is. Cacao, the bean from which chocolate is made, is actually one of the most nutrient dense foods on the planet, with over 1,500 active phytochemicals present.

Most of us know that there is something about chocolate that makes us feel better almost instantly. Well, that isn't just a psychological effect. There are two amazing compounds in chocolate that almost instantly affect our brain chemistry. The first is a compound called *anandamide*. This amazing substance actually binds to the same receptors in the brain as the psychoactive substance, THC, found in cannabis. As such, anandamide offers some similar properties, in that it evokes euphoria and also enhances clear creative thinking. It has been nicknamed "The Bliss Molecule".

Chocolate also contains a second substance called *phenylethylamine (PEA)*. This is another neurotransmitter that has been linked with elevation of mood and enhanced focus and clarity. This particular chemical is released in the nervous system when we first fall in love and have that euphoric feeling when everything is good in the world.

Lavender – is one of the best known plants for mood regulation. The fragrant oils that give lavender its distinctive aroma have a very mild but notable sedative effect upon the nervous system. It helps to calm and centre the mind, without causing excessive drowsiness.

Rose – is one of my favourite herbs for any kind of nervous system issue, especially when there is anxiety and depression present. The compound geraniol delivers a mild antidepressant effect upon the nervous system. It isn't 100 per cent clear why or how this happens, but it is likely to be a reflex effect that causes a general relaxation of the central nervous system.

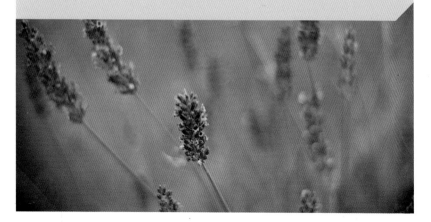

Omega Mania
Ice Lollies

Seeing as we were on the "sweet treats" theme,
I thought I would add this recipe for good measure.

1 large carton of organic plain live yogurt
2 handfuls of mixed berries
5 tablespoons flaxseed oil
2 teaspoons honey

* Add all the ingredients to a food processor, and blend into a smooth purée. Transfer the mixture to ice-lolly moulds and freeze. Enjoy as a sweet treat to bump up your omega 3 levels at any time.

MEDICINAL PROPERTIES

Flaxseed Oil – is an incredibly dense source of the vitally important omega 3 fatty acids. If you recall from the beginning of this section, omega 3 fatty acids are incredibly important for nerve cell health. This is because when these fats are metabolized, one of the end products, DHA, is the primary structural material used to lay down fresh myelin sheath – vital for the correct functioning of nerve cells and the carrying of their electrical signalling. This delicate membrane is constantly being broken down and rebuilt, so it is essential to obtain every day a good dietary source of the base structural material used for its renewal.

▶ Top Ingredients for Nervous System Health

Raw Seeds and Nuts – are rich sources of omega 3 and omega 6 fatty acids, vital for maintaining the structure and health of nerve cells.

Green Vegetables – are very rich in the mineral magnesium, vital for normal communication across and between nerve cells.

Whole Grains – such as brown rice, are very rich in B vitamins, which work to produce neurotransmitters in the brain and nervous system.

Bananas – rich in potassium, help to support healthy nerve function, and nerve communication.

▶ General Tips for Nervous System Health

▶ **Take time out.** If you feel as if the world and everyone in it is starting to get on top of you, it's time to take a break. Even if it is a five-minute walk around the block or ten minutes of meditation or focused relaxation. Our nervous system has the capacity to withstand a huge amount, provided that we give it the chance to recover. Continual stress and emotional upset can lead us to a state of nervous exhaustion, which can lead to serious burnout and even the onset of depression. Finding your own ways to cope with what life throws at you can literally be a lifesaver.

▶ **Reduce alcohol intake** as this can only bring you down. Alcohol, even though it can bring on the giggles, is a natural depressant. It affects brain chemistry in such a way that our "feel good" neurotransmitters, such as serotonin, become depleted.

▶ **Keep blood sugar even** as this can have a huge impact on both our mood and how we respond to stress. When we consume foods that send our blood sugar levels up too quickly, it throws our whole hormonal system out of balance. We get huge surges of insulin produced, in order to deal with the sudden rise in sugar. This causes disruption in the production and levels of other hormones throughout the body, and can lead to very low moods, and a feeling of being overwhelmed by the smallest of situations.

5

Nature's Edible Pharmacy

●

THIS SECTION OF THE BOOK delivers a simple A–Z guide to the most powerful, common medicinal foods on the planet. You will find that some obvious foods in the sequence are not included. This is because there are some foods that are very powerful from a purely nutritional perspective, such as oranges and their vitamin C content. The focus of this book is the foods that are powerful for reasons that stretch far beyond the scope of mere nutrition. Foods included are those that possess some powerful phytochemicals that make the foods more than just sources of fuel and nutrients, but make them medicines in their own right.

I have included a breakdown of the phytochemical content and medicinal properties for each food, plus some suggestions as to how they may be used.

Get in that kitchen, get creative, and cook yourself a cure!

Fruit

Fruit has to be a gift from the Gods, and is absolutely the single most important food for human beings. Do you think it is any coincidence that nature designed fruits to be so attractive to virtually all of our senses? Their colours are bright and vibrant. Their aromas are lingering, and their flavours are sweet and sensuous. They are our Number One food. Fruits are dense in antioxidants, minerals, and many of the water-soluble vitamins. They provide huge amounts of fibre, sustained energy, and take virtually no energy or effort to digest. Many fruits are also powerful medicines. Gone are the days when your medicine needs to taste awful. Make the most of nature's most divine of medicines.

Apples

We are all familiar with that age old saying, "An apple a day keeps the doctor away." How true that is! We could be forgiven for overlooking apples as being a medicinal food. They are such a simple everyday staple that we really do take them for granted. Simple though they may be, apples are a wonderful medicine.

One of the most important compounds found in apples is a soluble fibre called *pectin*. Those of you who make your own jams may well be familiar with pectin. It forms a gelatinous texture, helping jams to set. In the body, pectin has the ability to chemically bind to LDL cholesterol and carry it out of the body, via the digestive tract. Pectin is also known to support digestive transit, as it swells in the digestive tract, increasing bulk of the stool, and making the stool softer and easier to pass.

Apples have also gained a strong traditional reputation as a useful remedy for preventing asthma attacks. This folk remedy has now been backed up by a certain degree of scientific study. Almost every variety of apple contains significant levels of a flavonoid called *phloridzin*, which is known to help reduce localized inflammation of the bronchioles. Asthma is, after all, an immune-mediated reactive inflammation of the bronchioles, so any natural protection against this reaction is certainly going to aid the condition.

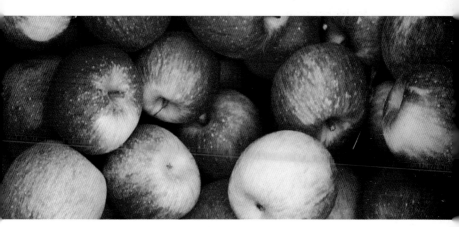

The final compound that is found in quite high levels in apples is a powerful chemical called *ellagic acid*. This magical antioxidant compound is known to be a powerful antimutagenic. This means that it is able to reduce the ability of potentially carcinogenic substances that initiate potentially cancerous changes in a cell's DNA. When certain environmental influences bind to a cell, or gain entry to a cell, they have the potential to change the genetic material within the cell's DNA, and that can lead to a sudden out-of-control cellular division that can be the start of a tumour.

▶ **Best way to use**
In general, I would say eaten whole and fresh. In some circumstances they can be cooked. Cooking will destroy some of the antioxidants, but will retain the pectin. I have included a recipe for Apple Jacks on page 64.

Bananas

One of the most widely consumed foods on the planet, the humble banana is more than just a sweet treat.

Bananas are famous for their incredibly high levels of the mineral potassium. This makes them an ideal food for the health of the cardiovascular system. This is because potassium is key in regulating the heart rhythm and the levels of body fluids. If levels of potassium are slightly higher than sodium, for example, our body will hold onto a lot less fluid. This is very beneficial for our blood pressure, because, the more fluid that the body holds onto, the more blood volume increases. As blood volume increases, simple physics tells us that the pressure within the vessels will also increase.

Bananas also contain a very sticky, soothing carbohydrate that has been traditionally used as a remedy for issues such as gastritis. It seems to soothe inflamed surfaces within the gastro intestinal tract.

▶ **Best way to use**
Raw bananas are great eaten whole or mashed with a little honey and mixed seeds. Yum!

Blueberries

Blueberries have become one of the most talked about and completely over-hyped foods on planet earth. These luscious, purple, little treats, are definitely one of the kings of the fruit domain, but have sadly been given an almost mythical reputation.

The most noteworthy property of blueberries is their super high antioxidant capacity. The vivid blue/purple pigment found in blueberry skins is given by a group of chemicals called *anthocyanidins*. These are the same family of chemicals that are found in grapes and red wine, and offer the health benefits associated with them. Anthocyanidins are essentially antioxidants first and foremost. This means that they help to protect tissues against oxidative damage. This is the kind of damage that is caused by normal metabolic reactions to energy production, or even chemical damage (think cigarette smoke and alcohol). This type of damage is associated with almost every disease at some level or another, from normal ageing, through to the initiation of cancer and heart disease. It is for this reason that high consumption of foods rich in antioxidants is associated with a reduced incidence of such diseases.

▶ **Best way to use**
Eaten with a little yogurt. The fats in the yogurt increase the absorption of the antioxidant chemicals.

Cherries

These delicious treats are easily one of my favourite fruits. The rich juicy flesh is bursting with antioxidants. The darker the cherries the better, as this represents higher levels of antioxidants.

Cherries are most famously used as a remedy for gout. This painful condition arises from crystals of uric acid forming in the joints. This causes spikes of uric acid crystal to press into surrounding soft tissues in the joint, which causes pain and triggers inflammation. Cherries contain a certain type of anthocyanidin (similar chemical to that found in red wine), unique to this fruit, which has been shown to inhibit a substance called *xanthine oxidase*, which is the enzyme that the body uses to manufacture uric acid. Inhibiting this enzyme will cause uric acid levels in the body to drop, and will reduce the likelihood of an excess starting to crystallize in the joints.

▶ **Best way to use**
Eaten fresh ideally. Can also be consumed as a pre-prepared concentrated juice.

Cranberries

Cranberries are synonymous with Christmas dinner, Thanksgiving, or a good Sunday roast. A close cousin to the blueberry, cranberries have a similarly high antioxidant level, coming from their deep red colour pigment.

In traditional medicine, cranberries are noted for their protective action against urinary tract infections. This is due to the presence of compounds called *proanthocyanidins*. These powerful antioxidants stop bacteria, such as *E. Coli*, from adhering to the inner wall of the urinary tract. For infection to occur, these bacteria must attach to the inner lining of the urinary tract. When this occurs, the immune system instigates its response, and inflammation occurs, which leads to

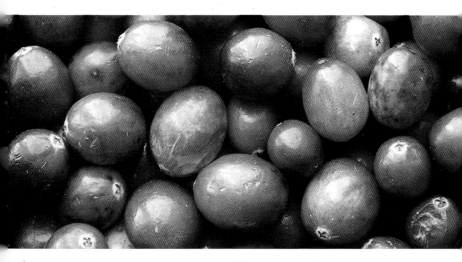

discomfort and the classical symptom of painful urination and urinary urgency. Preventing these bacteria adhering stops the infection. The proanthocyanidins in cranberry can also pluck them off the urinary tract walls if infection has already set in, thus drastically shortening duration of infection.

▶ **Best way to use**
I personally think that nothing can beat eating them fresh. They are quite sour, and are best mixed with a little yogurt. If you find the fresh berries disagreeable, then consuming the juice is OK, although definitely second place in my view.

Dates

I absolutely love dates (not just the dinner and flowers kind). They are like sweets to me. One of my favourite snacks to satisfy a sweet tooth is dates dipped in a little organic peanut butter.

Dates are a rich source of a special, large, and complex sugar, called *beta glucan*. This incredible sugar has some very profound health benefits. Firstly, it has a great reputation for removing LDL cholesterol from the body. It does this by chemically binding with it, rendering it inactive, and enabling it to be carried out of the body. The second, and probably most profound, effect of beta glucan is its ability to influence the immune system. It has been shown to cause a systemic rise in white blood cell numbers. It can actually cause the body, indirectly, to manufacture more white blood cells, and cause them to act in a far more aggressive manner. This effect has most famously been demonstrated in the medicinal mushrooms such as shiitake, maitake, and reishi. The beta glucans found in these mushrooms are the most biologically active and aggressive, but foods such as dates will still have this activity to a lesser degree.

▶ **Best way to use**
I tend to eat them just as they are or add them to things such as flapjacks.

Grapes

Grapes have always been associated with health and recovery. They seem to be the staple food taken into hospitals as a gift for sick friends and loved ones.

Grapes (red and purple variety) have probably gained their best reputation as a tool for protecting and maintaining heart health, especially in their fermented form (vino of course!). They contain a chemical pigment called *oligomeric proanthocyanidins*. These are part of the red/purple pigments in the grapes. These compounds are known to reduce the oxidization of LDL cholesterol, thus preventing arterial damage. It isn't actually cholesterol itself that causes damage to the circulatory system, rather the body oxidizing the cholesterol, which then causes inflammation, which in turn causes damage to the lining of the arteries, which then leads to blood clot formation.

Oligomeric proanthocyanidins have also been shown to cause a notable relaxation of the muscles that line the blood vessel walls. In doing so, they allow the blood vessel walls to widen, thus increasing their internal space. Simple physics tells us that, if the contents of the vessel (i.e. blood volume) stay the same, but the size of the vessel increases, the pressure within that vessel will, of course, go down.

Grapes also contain another compound believed to be linked to their cardioprotective properties. That is the antioxidant compound resveratrol. This compound is known to reduce the build-up of plaques within the artery walls, thus minimizing the risk of vascular injury, and the inevitable clot formation that follows this. Resveratrol is also reputed to be an anti-ageing ingredient for the skin. Best rely on the whole, raw grapes for this rather than the red wine. As with all things in life, there is always a trade off. There would be little point in having lovely wrinkle-free skin, if that was accompanied by a bright red boozer's nose, and eye bags that would make Miss Piggy look like a beauty queen!

▶ **Best way to use**

A glass of a good quality red wine with a meal is one of my ideas of heaven. Not only does this deliver some of the protective properties mentioned above, but alcohol acts as a potentiator. In

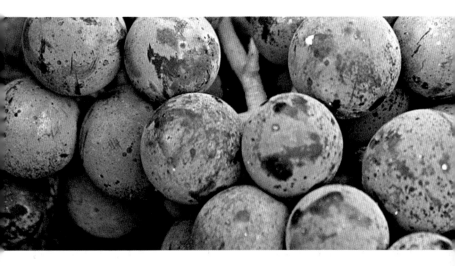

herbal medicine, we see alcohol as a substance that can drive the active chemicals in plants much deeper into the physiology. It basically makes the compounds more bioavailable to the body. However, wine shouldn't be over consumed. Once you move past 1–2 glasses a day, the protective properties are taken over by damage and irritation to the liver and upper digestive tract. So be sensible. The best way really is eat the grapes whole and fresh. But I guess we all need a little fun.

Lemons & Limes

I have included these two fruits together, as, aside from a couple of tiny insignificant chemicals, they are virtually identical. Lemons certainly have to be one of the most widely consumed fruits on the planet. Limes are responsible for the discovery of vitamin C. When British sailors went out to sea on long journeys, most would end up suffering from the deficiency condition of scurvy. It was observed eventually that expeditions that carried limes on board for consumption would have no episodes of scurvy whatsoever. This eventually led to the discovery of vitamin C. This also led to us Brits earning the unfortunate nickname of limeys!

Both lemons and limes have a very high concentration of a compound called *kaempferol*. This substance is known to be a powerful protective agent against cancer, as it is known to reduce uncontrolled cell division. It seems most protective, at least from an epidemiological perspective, against breast cancer.

Kaempferol is also a potent antibiotic agent. This was first demonstrated in village populations in West Africa, where there was frequent and aggressive cholera outbreak. Lime juice was added to their staple rice-based dish, and episodes of cholera began to decline. This led to further investigation that revealed that kaempferol was the magic bullet in this case.

Lemons and limes also offer further cancer protective activity, thanks to the presence of a powerful phytochemical called *limonin*. Limonin is believed to be chemoprotective. This means that it is able to defend cells against the damaging effects of carcinogens. Carcinogens are chemical compounds, both natural metabolic by products and environmental chemicals, that can cause damage to a cell's DNA, which may then lead to an unnatural division and cancerous changes of the cell.

▶ **Best way to use**
Add fresh lemon or lime juice to salad dressings, dips, sauces, or to hot water.

Mango

Mangoes are one of my favourite fruits. I'm actually eating an ice cold one from the fridge as I write this. They are sweet, aromatic, and so very exotic.

Apart from being very high in the antioxidant compound beta carotene, they are also a useful digestive aid. Similar to the papaya, mangoes contain some highly active enzymes that are beneficial in the correct digestion of proteins. These enzymes are so powerful that mango is sometimes used as a meat tenderizer.

▶ **Best way to use**
Eaten fresh, or blended with natural yogurt and a little water to make a refreshing mango lassi.

Papaya

Papaya is a very delicious sweet fruit. Not one of my particular favourites, but it certainly satisfies the sweet craving from time to time.

Papaya contains some very powerful enzymes. The most well known of these is a compound called *papain*. This is a powerful protein-digesting enzyme. I often recommend papaya, or an extract of papain, to individuals who have had long-standing illness or are weak and need building up, as it increases their protein digestion and absorption. Papain is also commonly used for allergies, especially hay fever. This is because it is believed to be an effective natural antihistamine. In allergic reactions such as hay fever, there is a localized histamine release that is responsible for most of the inflammation and symptoms associated with such conditions. Anything that can manage the levels of histamine produced can have a notable effect upon the severity of such conditions.

▶ **Best way to use**
Eaten raw, juiced, or taken as an extract.

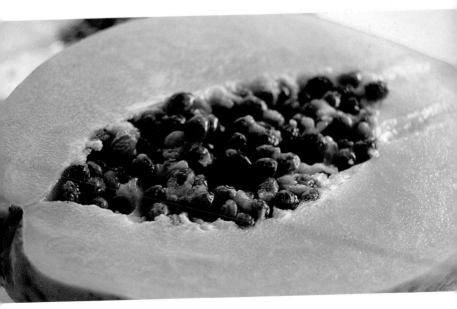

Pineapple

Another of my favourite fruits. Pineapples conjure up images in my mind of white sandy beaches and grass skirts. Maybe that's just me! But their exotic flavour and aroma is certainly comforting on some level.

Pineapples contain a very powerful enzyme called *bromelain*. This wonderful compound is great for enhancing protein digestion, but its medicinal properties are far more profound than that. Bromelain is a very powerful anti-inflammatory. It can rapidly and efficiently soften swollen tissues, and ease them back to normal functioning. I find pineapple to be a very useful food for arthritics, and those with inflammatory issues of the digestive tract.

▶ **Best way to use**

I tend to juice pineapple more often than anything else. It is also great in smoothies too. The most important thing to note, however you choose to eat it, is to ensure that you do not discard the slightly tougher inner core of the pineapple. This contains the highest concentration of bromelain.

Grains

Grains have, without doubt, become one of the single main staple foods on the planet. Virtually every culture has grains at the forefront of its diet: the rice in Asia, the maize in Africa and South America, and wheat in Europe and North America. Grains are an important part of the human food chain.

These staple foods can at once be some of the most health-promoting foods around, and the most detrimental to our health. The problem arose when we began the process of refining. Refining grains mostly involves the removal of the outer coating of the grain. This is the difference between white rice and brown rice, for example. It's the same grain, just one has the outer husk left on, and one doesn't.

The refining of grains creates some significant problems. Firstly, much of the nutrition and phytochemistry is found in the outer husk. This means that the refined grains are essentially supplying dead calories, and in cultures where these foods are a real dietary staple, means that a population can really become deficient in important nutrients.

The second, and in my opinion, most significant, issue that arises from refining foods is the impact that these foods have on our blood sugar. When the grains are in the original (whole) state, they release their sugars into the bloodstream at a very slow rate. This gives us a nice stable energy level. This slow release doesn't upset our blood sugar in any way, and our body can use the sugar properly, over a long period of time, as it is coming in at a constant trickle. However, when the grains are refined, they cause a sudden and very sharp rise in blood sugar levels. This makes the body release a large amount of insulin (the hormone that regulates the amount of sugar in our bloodstream), in order to deal with the sudden rise in blood sugar. Insulin forces the body's cells to "suck in" the sugar as quickly as possible, to get it out of the bloodstream. However, the cells can only take so much sugar in at one time and, very often, when consuming refined carbohydrates, there is still an excess in circulation. In this case, the next method that the body employs to remove the excess sugar is to turn it into fat, so it can be stored as body fat to get it out of the way.

Refined carbohydrate consumption has been directly linked to diseases such as heart disease, cancer, type 2 diabetes, and obesity. I believe that our consumption of refined carbohydrates (think white bread, white pasta, white rice, sugar in tea, etc) is one of the most significant contributing factors to the increase in disease in our modern times.

Amaranth

Amaranth is not a widely known grain in the Western world. It is a tiny grain that once became a staple food for the Aztecs.

Aside from being a gluten-free grain, rich in protein and every conceivable mineral on earth, amaranth has a track record as being an effective astringent, for use in digestive problems such as excessive diarrhoea. Astringents are essentially plants that help to "dry out" secretory surfaces – such as those that line the gut. They do this by irritating those surfaces, causing them to release proteins that essentially develop a lining on such surfaces, preventing their secretory action. In the context of diarrhoea, the astringent action of amaranth stops too much water entering the digestive tract too rapidly, so helps to give more bulk and texture to the stool.

The most interesting thing about amaranth, however, is its impact upon cholesterol. Something in this grain, yet to be identified, increases the liver's production of an enzyme called *7-alpha-hydroxylase*. This is the enzyme that the liver uses to break down cholesterol into bile acids, which can then be easily excreted via the bowel.

▶ **Best way to use**
    As a replacement for rice. Boil until soft.

Brown Rice

Associated with health food and healthy eating. Mention brown rice to most people, and images of beards and sandals soon arise. One of the absolute staple foods, rice, when prepared in the right way, can be one of the most health-giving foods around. I remember, from my time out in Japan, eating brown rice at least twice a day, my energy levels and digestion were fantastic, and my appetite sustained. This glorious grain is now a common inclusion into my diet.

Brown rice is rich in a whole host of compounds that can help to lower cholesterol. These range from simple dietary fibres, through to

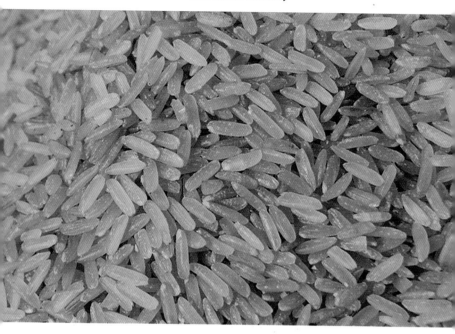

more complex phytochemicals. The most interesting of these is a compound called *gamma-oryzanol*. This compound is well known to reduce the production of LDL cholesterol.

Brown rice also contains a large amount of a group of antioxidant compounds called *polyphenols*. These antioxidant phytochemicals help to protect the inner lining of the blood vessels against damage.

Aside from this, the amazing fibre content of brown rice makes it a wonderful food for diabetics, and anyone wanting to balance out their blood sugar. This is because it is in itself a very slow release sugar food. However, its fibre also slows down the release of the sugars from other foods consumed with it. This means that the meal will not cause rapid rises in blood sugar or the inevitable insulin spike that follows.

▶ **Best way to use**
I tend to use brown rice with curries and the usual dishes that would suit a rice accompaniment. However, it is possible to use the rice flour to make gluten-free pasta and bread.

Buckwheat

Buckwheat is another grain that is not that well known, but is becoming very popular. Eaten widely in Asian countries, such as Japan, it is often ground into a flour to make noodles and pastas.

Buckwheat is incredibly high in a group of antioxidant compounds called *flavonoids*. Two in particular, rutin and quercetin, really stand out. Rutin has, in clinical trials, been shown to offer significant protection against damage to the inner lining of blood vessels and clot formation. Quercetin, on the other hand, is an incredibly powerful compound that is useful against allergies. During the allergic response, certain white blood cells release a chemical called *histamine*, which causes a localized inflammatory response. It is the action of histamine that causes many of the symptoms of issues such as hay fever. Quercetin seems to, somehow, inhibit the release of histamine at this local level, so can offer significant improvement in some allergic symptoms.

Both rutin and quercetin have also been associated with a reduction in platelet aggregation. This means that they play a role in protecting us against excessive blood clotting, which helps prevent heart attacks and strokes.

▶ **Best way to use**
Buckwheat grains are fantastic toasted and used in breakfast cereals. The most commonly eaten form of buckwheat, though, is soba noodles. These Japanese noodles are heavenly stir fried with vegetables or served cold with a sweet soy and wasabi dip.

Oats

Oats are among the most widely consumed grains in the world. They are a breakfast staple in Europe and the US, and have been associated with health for decades. But what exactly is so special about them?

Oats contain a soluble fibre known as beta glucan. This complex sugar forms a gelatinous type texture in the digestive tract. In this state, it can physically bind to LDL cholesterol, and carry it out of the digestive tract to prevent it being absorbed into the bloodstream.

Beta glucan also has a very interesting influence on the immune system. It has been shown in numerous trials to stimulate the production of a group of immune cells called *natural killer cells*. It does this by having an interaction with patches of tissue in the gut wall called *Peyer's patches*. These patches of tissue are basically like surveillance stations, watching what is happening inside the gut. These patches contain a lot of immune cells that tell the rest of the immune system what to do if an invader is making its way into the body via the gut. These cells do this by sending chemical messengers throughout the body in order to recruit the correct type of immune cells for the invader they have come across. Beta glucan fools the cells in the Peyer's patches that the body is under a specific type of bacterial attack, and causes them to encourage the production of more white blood cells. This response, in short, can strengthen the immune system in times of infection and stress. It is beta glucan that makes medicinal mushrooms such as shiitake and maitake such powerhouses (although the mushrooms contain far higher levels).

Oats have always been traditionally used in Western herbal medicine as a "nervine tonic", specifically for nervous exhaustion. They seem to have a deeply relaxing and restorative quality on the nervous system. Exactly why this would be the case remains unclear. It may be, at least in part, due to the high levels of B vitamins in oats, as these nutrients are very relaxing and regulating for the nervous system.

▶ **Best way to use**
Few things are more comforting than a bowl of warm porridge on a winter's morning. This is one of the best ways to serve oats, as the heat encourages the release of the beta glucan (this is what makes it go all thick and gloopy). I always advise making porridge with water rather than milk, as the proteins in milk can actually bind to the beta glucan and hinder its absorption by the body.

Nuts and Seeds

There has certainly been somewhat of an upward trend in the regular consumption of nuts and seeds in recent years. Fifteen years ago, the only contact most of us would have with these foods is the odd one turning up in a cereal bar or breakfast muesli, or the scattering of sesame seeds on the top of a burger bun! In the last few years, however, countless nutrition and lifestyle books, health experts, and press articles, have enlightened us to the nutritional power that these foods have. Beyond their mere nutritional profile, of a rich source of omega 3 and 6 fatty acids, plus a few minerals, some nuts and seeds have some pretty powerful medicinal phytochemicals present too!

Apricot Kernels

Often overlooked as a seed, but a seed indeed. These wonderful foods have caused great controversy in recent times, due to their potential properties. The kernels that are most commonly sold in health food stores are of the bitter variety, although sweet ones are available. It is the bitter variety that has the beneficial effects, and the bitter flavour is an indicator of the active constituent.

The most widely publicized compound that apricot kernels contain is an interesting compound called *amygdalin* – otherwise known as B17. This compound is made up of a whole array of chemicals, including the poison cyanide. This sounds rather dramatic, but is believed to be really quite harmless under normal circumstances. When it is bound within amygdalin, cyanide is inactive because specific enzymes, which are required to release it from its bonds, are not present in healthy cells. However, research is indicating that cancerous cells do have the enzymes necessary for releasing cyanide. When a cell becomes cancerous, there are changes in the cell's DNA which causes it to behave in an irregular fashion. This includes the manufacture and activity of unique enzymes. When the enzymes begin to work upon amygdalin, the cyanide component of this

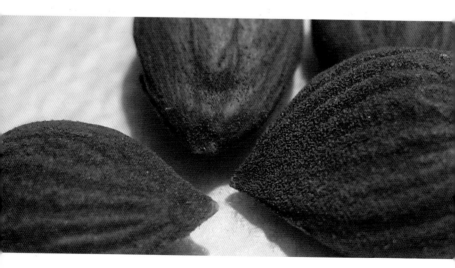

compound is activated. As cyanide is a potent cellular poison, it causes the cell it is within to die. It is worth bearing in mind that these claims still remain theoretical. What is clear, however, is that there has been an array of positive clinical trials using apricot kernels and B17 in the treatment of cancer. B17 is also a very powerful antioxidant compound, providing all the usual benefits associated with such compounds. This will also provide added protection against the formation of cancerous changes in cells. Much of these findings are thanks to the work of Dr Ernst T Krebs who claimed, "If a person would eat seven to ten apricot kernels a day for life, then barring Chernobyl, he is likely to be cancer free". It is worthwhile to note, that it is only the bitter variety of this apricot that should be chosen as it is the amygdalin that gives them their bitter taste.

▶ **Best way to use**

It is recommended by the UK Food Standards Agency that no more than 3–4 kernels be eaten a day, so just eating them as a mid-morning snack can be ideal.

Brazil Nuts

Brazil nuts are one of my absolute favourites. There is just something about their luscious creamy flavour that most people adore. These nuts aren't necessarily high in any exotic phytochemicals, but I felt them worthy of inclusion, because they are a great food for immunity, and for managing inflammation. This is because they are exceptionally high in the trace mineral selenium. This potent mineral helps the body to produce its own natural antioxidant enzyme, called *glutathione peroxidase*. This helps assist the body in the breakdown and clearance of waste products from the body. It also helps to regulate the activity of certain groups of white blood cells, so can improve immune function, particularly in inflammatory conditions.

▶ **Best way to use**

I love to make a nut pâté out of them, or include them in veggie burgers, or just munch them straight from the bag.

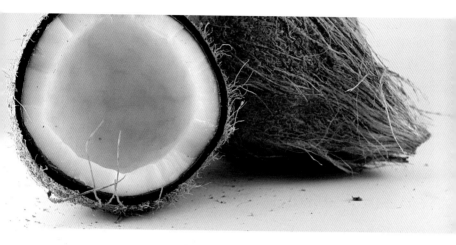

Coconut

Yes, that's right... it's a nut.

Coconut has some wonderful nutritional and medicinal properties. The water within coconuts is the best isotonic drink on the planet. It contains the perfect balance of the electrolytes used by our body – sodium, calcium, potassium, and magnesium. It can rehydrate in minutes.

Coconuts also contain a very unique type of fat, called *medium chain triglycerides* (*MCTs*), which are believed to aid in weight loss, due to their ability to force dietary fats into being burnt as energy, rather than used as a storage medium. On a personal note, I always get a little suspicious when I hear of "miracle" weight loss claims for anything, so for me, the jury is still out.

Coconuts also contain a compound called *lauric acid*, which appears to offer some considerable potential benefits as an antiviral agent. When we take in a source of lauric acid, our body converts it into a substance called *monolaurin*. This compound can be very protective against all manner of viruses. It works by breaking down certain structures on the outside of fatty coated viruses. In particular, it attacks the structures that viruses use to attach to and enter our cells. Without this ability, the viruses cannot cause infection, cannot replicate, and quickly die out.

Coconut is also very high in another acid called *caprylic acid*. This is one of the best things for dealing with Candida infection of the digestive tract. Caprylic acid can cause Candida to die almost on contact.

▶ **Best way to use**
I use the oil in dishes almost every day. It is great for curries and sweet dishes because of its wonderful flavour. Coconut milk is also a great addition to smoothies, and coconut flesh is wonderful in desserts and sweet, raw food recipes.

Flaxseeds (linseed)

Flaxseeds are definitely one of the staple features of any health food shop shelf. Traditionally, flax has been used as a gentle laxative as it has a semi soluble outer coating that forms a gelatinous mass, which can help "move things along" a little. They are also a rich source of omega 3 fatty acids, offering an alternative to oily fish for vegetarians.

The most interesting thing, in my opinion, about flaxseeds, is their content of a group of compounds called *plant lignans*. Lignans are a type of fibre that is known to bind to oestrogen receptors on the surfaces of cells. This binding is believed to offer protection against some hormone dependant cancers such as breast cancer. Lignans also help to break down and remove oestrogen from the body, by increasing the production of chemicals that facilitate this in the body.

▶ **Best way to use**
On cereals, in smoothies, in crackers and breads, or taken in a small glass of water.

Pumpkin Seeds

These seemingly ordinary little seeds are actually medicinal powerhouses. I love them. Raw, roasted, eaten straight from the bag, or made into a "butter", I'll eat them any way that they come.

Pumpkin seeds have long been known as a perfect food for prostate health. This is because they contain a compound called *beta sitosterol*, which actually helps to inhibit normal testosterone turning into its evil twin – dihydrotestosterone. In the prostate, normal testosterone is conducive to the overall health and normal functioning of the prostate. However, certain circumstances can cause this healthy testosterone to be turned into an aggressively mischievous version called *dihydrotestosterone*, which can cause enlargement of the prostate, which can be the starting point for prostatic cancer.

Beta sitosterol is also highly beneficial to heart health. This is because it helps to reduce cholesterol. You may well be aware of the myriad of drinks and spreads, loaded with "plant sterols" that reduce cholesterol. Well, beta sitosterol is one of the most powerful of the plant sterols. Essentially, these compounds help to block the absorption of cholesterol in the intestines. When our liver manufactures cholesterol, a large proportion is actually released into the intestine from the liver where it is reabsorbed back into the bloodstream where it can do its work. Blocking this intestinal absorption has been shown to notably reduce blood cholesterol levels.

Pumpkin seeds also contain another powerful chemical called *cucurbitin*. Cucurbitin is a major constituent in these seeds and has been shown to have a very powerful anti-parasitic effect in many test tube studies. This gives pumpkin seeds the potential to be used as remedies against such digestive issues as Candida, and maybe as an adjunct in the treatment of food poisoning.

▶ **Best way to use**

Use raw whenever possible as the cooking process can seriously damage the beneficial fats that these seeds contain. I like to use them in pâtés, salads, or eaten whole as a snack.

Culinary Herbs and Spices

Many of us today are becoming increasingly familiar with the huge array of exotic spices and aromatic herbs that the world has to offer. Our love of fancy food and exotic flavours has led us along a path of culinary discovery as far as herbs and spices are concerned. Sadly, many of us think that the journey ends there. We think that herbs and spices are little gifts from nature, merely designed to add a little pleasure and zing to our food. This is, in fact, just the very beginning. Herbs and spices are some of the most powerful medicinal compounds on earth. Some are equally as strong as pharmaceutical drugs, and all of them are immeasurably safer. So revered were many of these herbs and spices that they were actually used as a form of currency in some ancient cultures – particularly ancient Greece and Egypt.

The fact is that herbs and spices have been a focal part of traditional medicinal systems for millennia. The Ayurvedic traditional medicine system of India, with over 5,000 years of wisdom, makes full use of the many exotic spices found on India's shores. Likewise with Thai traditional medicine, where many culinary recipes double as folk remedies for many ailments. Traditional Chinese medicine also has many of the more common culinary herbs as medicines and ingredients for traditional herbal preparations.

For some illogical reason, modern Western society now views medicinal herbs and spices as some kind of New Age hogwash, that, while sounding nice, have no substance or scientific grounding. Nothing could be further from the truth. The chemistry of the aromatic plants is among some of the most complex and highly active in nature. They are the strongest medicines of all plants. The substances that deliver their enticing smells and exotic flavours are the very same that can have all kinds of incredible interactions with our body tissues and systems. Some are powerful antibiotics, some are painkillers, and others can tackle inflammation.

This section will take you through these amazing plants one by one and demonstrate just how effective they are, not to mention giving you some inspiration to get in the kitchen and get creative with nature's most powerful and pleasant medicines.

Aniseed

This sweet and aromatic spice is recognizable to almost everyone, and has been a sweetshop favourite for centuries. In the same family as celery, fennel, dill, and carrots, aniseed has been used in traditional remedies in Europe since the fourteenth century, across many countries. The fragrant oil anethol, the substance that gives the instantly recognizable smell, is responsible for the medicinal actions of this plant. The oil has the ability, once ingested, to relax smooth muscle surfaces that it comes into contact with. Smooth muscle is the muscle that makes up the walls of tissues such as blood vessels and the digestive tract. This muscle is laid down in several layers that run in differing directions, so that when they contract or relax, they alter the shape and diameter of the organ that they compose. This contraction and relaxation regulates the normal functioning of the organ in question. Ingesting plants that can have an effect on this musculature can literally manipulate normal functioning to give a therapeutic effect.

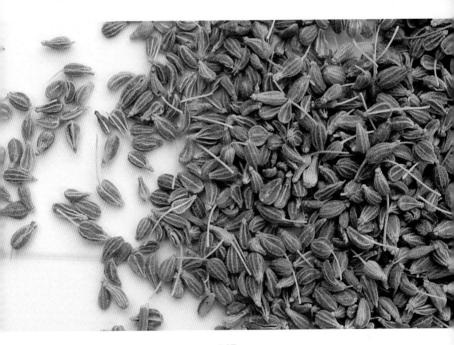

Aniseed is traditionally used in tea form as an antispasmodic for the intestines. This means that, due to the actions described above, it can relieve the strong, spasm-like pain associated with conditions such as IBS and colic. The wonderful fragrant essential oils are able to relax smooth muscle of the intestinal walls, thus easing such excessive spasms – which are, in fact, just a more forceful and rapid manifestation of our normal intestinal contractions peristalsis. Aniseed is also considered an effective carminative. This means that it is able to disperse gas within the digestive system, thus making it an excellent remedy for any type of bloating and digestive discomfort, and proves especially useful in infant colic, Candida infection, and IBS.

Aniseed has also been used as a traditional cough remedy. Its traditional preparation was infusion into spirits or wine, to make a tonic liquor called *Anisette*. This remedy has been thought to open up the small tubes (bronchioles) of the lungs, and ease bronchitis and asthma. If the bronchioles are dilated and widened, it makes it far easier to cough up or move phlegm, not to mention increasing airflow. The seed was also ground and used in lozenges to ease mild coughs. This allows the herb to gently coat the area and act for longer.

▶ **Best ways to use**
For digestive complaints, tea or any kind of water infusion is the best method for rapid results. I would recommend 2–3 teaspoons of seeds, gently crushed with the back of a spoon, per person, per cup.

Basil

This vibrant green staple of Italian cuisine is familiar to us all, and is one of the easiest home remedies to obtain or to grow. It is also one of the easiest to use, as it can be added directly to your food in a million and one different ways. Used as medicine all over the world, basil has a history of medicinal use in traditional Chinese medicine spanning more than 3,000 years. Its use in European medicine most likely spans a similar time frame.

Being in the same family as mint, basil shares some of the same properties. As a result, basil is a useful remedy for bloating, digestive cramps, flatulence, and colic. As with many fragrant spices, it is the potent fragrant oils found within that have a relaxing effect on the musculature of the intestinal wall, easing cramps and spasms.

Basil is also an effective anxiolytic (calms anxiety) and sedative, so is a tasty stress-relief aid. Many traditional texts have made the recommendation of basil tea for mild depression and melancholy. This traditional application, however, is not well supported in modern herbal literature, so its effectiveness remains unclear.

The action of basil that interests me the most, however, is its anthelmintic/vermifuge activity. These old medical terms refer to a remedy that has the ability to rid the body of parasites such as yeasts and worms. In today's society of convenience foods and high sugar intake, the presence of parasites, particularly yeasts such as *Candida albicans* is a very common problem. It is therefore reassuring that there are foodstuffs that we can consume (along with getting our diet right in the first place) to aid our body's defence against these troublesome parasites. Again, the powerful essential oils present in basil are believed to be responsible for this action. Such oils can be really quite toxic to more simple organisms and kill them off rapidly. The key to this application, however, is to make sure that the foodstuff is not cooked so as to gain the main benefit.

▶ **Best way to use**
The good thing about basil is its versatility. It can be used in so many dishes. However, I'd recommend, for maximum effect, that you use this ingredient raw where possible, in order to preserve its essential oils. See page 36 for a wonderful pesto recipe!

Cardamom

This is one of my favourite medicinal spices. Hailing from India, its beautiful flavour and aroma lend itself well to both sweet and savoury dishes, not to mention herbal preparations, traditional to this country.

Cardamom is commonly used as a digestive aid in many traditional medical systems, again due to the presence of some powerful fragrant essential oils that have the properties outlined above, making it another remedy to consider in digestive complaints such as nausea, bloating, and digestive cramps.

There is, however, one therapeutic use of cardamom that is unique among the spices, and that is as an aid in the treatment of mild depression and melancholy. There is a large amount of empirical evidence around to support this, and I have also observed this effect in clinical practice. However, clinical trial data is very limited at present. It is believed that compounds in cardamom may interact with serotonin receptors in the digestive tract. Serotonin is a neurotransmitter (communication and signalling molecule produced by the nervous system) that is associated with mood elevation and a more relaxed state. It is thought that some of the chemistry of cardamom may actually bind to serotonin receptors within the walls of the digestive tract, and cause a rise in this neurotransmitter to occur throughout the body. It is important to remain aware that this is still a theory at present and that more data needs to be acquired. What is a certainty is that cardamom works – somehow!

▶ **Best way to use**
Cardamom is amazing in teas, or used in desserts. My favourite tea is cardamom, skullcap, lavender and rose.

Chilli

This powerful fiery spice that gives curries their fire has been used in almost every culture in one way or another for both culinary and medicinal purposes. It is indeed a very versatile medicine, with its effects spanning many body systems and physical conditions and situations.

One of the major applications of chilli is as a cardiovascular tonic that enhances circulation. The powerful chemical capsaicin, that gives chilli its fiery flavour, has a very potent effect on the musculature of artery walls. In short, it almost forces a relaxation of the arterial walls via irritating the smooth muscle causing it to suddenly relax, thus widening the blood vessels and enhancing circulation – especially to the peripheries (fingers, toes, and brain). Another positive consequence of this action is that blood pressure is lowered – the vessel has widened, so its internal diameter increases, putting less pressure on the vessel wall, lessening the likelihood of injury.

Chilli is also a renowned painkiller when used topically (on the outer surfaces). When it is applied in this manner to a painful area, it has an instant initial irritating effect on the nerve endings of surrounding tissues. This irritating effect increases the release of the pain-signalling chemical known as "substance P". Now, this may sound somewhat counter intuitive to increase the production of a nerve-signalling compound that signals pain, but, the ingenious action of capsaicin is to not only increase the release of substance P, but to block its re-uptake by the nerve. After applying capsaicin to the affected area a few times, the levels of substance P in the nerve endings of surrounding tissues have essentially been spent, so there is nothing left to send the pain signal to the brain. Isn't Mother Nature amazing?! Pain killing aside, topical application of chilli can have an immense stimulatory effect on circulation to that area. To this end, these two actions make it a perfect remedy for cold stiff arthritis.

Chilli is also gaining a reputation as a potential weight loss tool. While I don't like any "magic bullet" type claims being made for individual ingredients, it is useful to be aware of such things. Again it is the spicy compound capsaicin that is reputed to deliver these effects. One study carried out in Taiwan suggests that capsaicin may have the ability to destroy cells called *preadipocytes*. These are juvenile cells that eventually turn into fat cells. Other small-scale studies have revealed that taking an extract of capsaicin increases the overall metabolic rate in test subjects, with some significant weight loss observed.

▶ **Best way to use**

Chilli does need to be used with caution, as it is so irritating. It can be used in cooking to generate the internal stimulating effects described above. It can also be puréed and applied directly to the skin for pain relief. For best results, cover this purée with a plaster or bandage.

Cinnamon

I absolutely adore the taste of this spice and it is a regular feature in a lot of my cooking. I find it has a comforting and nurturing quality. It has been used as a medicine in both Eastern and Western cultures for hundreds of years and is very diverse in its applications.

The first application that comes to mind when I think of cinnamon is gentle stimulation of the circulatory system. It is most likely that it is the essential oils contained in cinnamon that have this effect. The likelihood is that these compounds have the ability to relax the musculature of the vessel walls, leading to an overall widening of the vessel. This is useful in issues such as cold hands and feet. I also find that cinnamon is particularly useful in painful menstrual cramps, where improved blood flow in the pelvic region can relieve the symptoms somewhat.

Cinnamon is also a powerful antifungal agent, especially for fungal infections of the digestive tract, such as Candidiasis. *Candida albicans* infection is something that is drastically on the rise in modern society. With our increased intake of convenience foods, high sugar snacks, alcohol, and yeasty breads, yeast infections of the gut are becoming more prominent and have been linked with food allergies, recurrent headaches, skin rashes, and fatigue, to name but a few ailments. The number one key to tackling this type of infection is adopting the correct diet and lifestyle, but there are herbs and remedies that can help. The powerful essential oils found in cinnamon contain active compounds called *cinnamaldehyde*, *cinnamyl acetate*, and *cinnamyl alcohol* that give it its potent antifungal properties. These oils are believed to kill fungi such as yeasts and Candida, on contact, causing them to die off, and slough off from the gut wall ready for expulsion via the bowel.

Cinnamon is now getting a considerable reputation as a blood sugar balancing agent that has proved to be useful in the management of type 2 diabetes. Type 2 diabetes is very different from the diabetes that individuals are born with, that requires a lifetime of self-administered insulin injections. It is a disease of modern living. Type

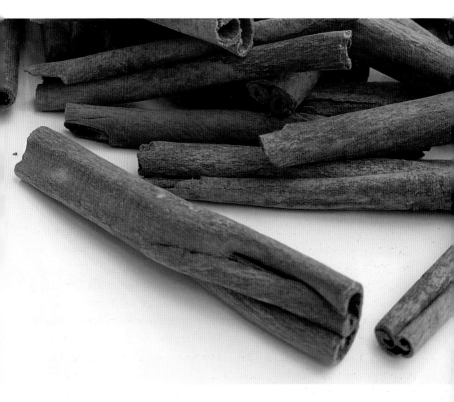

2 diabetes is essentially a state in which the cells of the body have started to ignore the signal of insulin. Insulin is released when our blood sugar rises up beyond a certain threshold level. Its job is to tell the cells of the body that they need to pull this sugar in, and convert it into a usable energy source. This message is received via receptors that line the outside of cells in body tissues. Once the cells receive the signal, they take action. Now, in type 2 diabetes, it is safe to assume that an individual's blood sugar has been getting very high, for a very long time. By very high, I mean the type of sugar rush that comes from eating sugary snacks, refined white carbohydrates, and excessive alcohol. In the initial stages, cell receptors listen to the constant signalling from insulin that arises from consuming such foods. However, after a while the cell receptors soon start to suspect that

something is awry. They start to wonder why there is so much insulin in circulation, and think that maybe the insulin has gone a little crazy and doesn't know quite what it is doing. Therefore they begin to ignore its message. As a result of this, the levels of blood sugar start to rise as less and less of it is pulled into the cells. It is at this stage that type 2 diabetes is diagnosed. It is believed that cinnamon has the ability to directly influence special structures on the outer surfaces of cells known as glucose transporters. These structures are used by cells to grab glucose from the blood and fluids that bathe the tissues, and pull it into the cells for conversion into energy. Studies suggest that cinnamon has the ability to increase the amount of these that are produced and how effectively they take glucose from the circulation into the cell.

▶ **Best way to use**
To tap into its blood sugar management properties, cinnamon really needs to be used quite liberally in cooking, and in smoothies, etc. Just a teaspoon or a shake of the powder would be insufficient. Cinnamon can also be consumed as a tea made from the dried bark. Prepared in this way it acts as a gentle warming circulatory stimulant.

Garlic

Garlic is one of the most powerful medicines on the entire planet, and its amazing properties could fill an entire book by itself. It is a remedy that has benefits for virtually every system in the body. Everyone is aware of the strong odour of garlic. It is this pungent and powerful aspect of the plant that is responsible for a large part of the medicinal properties of garlic. These compounds, also known as volatile factors, include the sulphur-based chemicals allicin, diallyl disulphide, and diallyl trisulphide to name but a few. Many of these chemicals become more active when garlic is crushed or chopped, as this starts an enzymatic process that releases more and more of these compounds. These pungent-smelling chemicals act as fabulous antibacterial and antiviral agents in the upper respiratory tract. They are not broken down by the body at all and are excreted from the body via, you guessed it, the breath (hence garlic's powerful antisocial properties). These powerful chemicals destroy bacteria and viruses as they rush through the airways on exhalation. These compounds are also extremely active in the digestive tract and have a fantastic localized effect upon any kind of nasty invader in the gut, such as the yeast infection *Candida albicans*. The oils are powerful enough to kill this simple yeast on contact, and aid in its removal from the body.

One of the properties of garlic that has been all over the world press for the last ten to fifteen years is the protective effects it has on the cardiovascular system. There are literally hundreds of studies that have shown that garlic is able to offer some protection against the formation of plaques within artery walls. It is also well established that regular garlic consumption can help to lower the production of LDL (bad) cholesterol, and increase the production of HDL (good) cholesterol. It is not 100 per cent clear how garlic manages to do this, but it may be in part due to interactions that it has with the liver – the cholesterol manufacturing plant. There are also some reported effects against high blood pressure. It is believed that garlic is a very effective vasodilator, meaning that it can cause blood vessels to relax, which helps to lower overall pressure inside the vessels.

The sulphurous compounds in garlic have also been shown to interact with certain enzymes that cause inflammation to occur. This interaction actually gives garlic some notable anti-inflammatory properties, when consumed regularly.

There is also some evidence to suggest that regular garlic consumption may offer protection against colon cancer. It is believed that it can prevent cells of the colon from damage (antimutagenic), and can also stop any cancerous cells from growing.

► **Best way to use**

All ways and every way. Garlic is nearly always best used raw when you can stand it. Raw in salad dressings, sprinkled over roasted vegetables, added to various dishes at the last minute. Consuming it raw keeps the active chemicals intact. Whole slices of garlic can also be placed over fungal nail infections, and secured with a plaster.

Ginger

This beautiful spice has been used in virtually every traditional healing system in the world, spanning millennia. It has been consumed in the traditional diets of almost every Asian country, and has become a very common ingredient in contemporary Western cookery too.

Ginger has been traditionally used for the treatment of stomach upsets such as nausea, morning sickness, and travel sickness. It is also a great carminative agent, meaning that it can disperse wind and intestinal bloating. Ginger is also a wonderful circulatory stimulant as it has the ability to relax the walls of the blood vessels, thus increasing blood flow. In this context it is a great remedy for cold extremities, and conditions such as Reynaud's disease, where circulation is greatly affected.

There is another exciting action that ginger offers, which is the one that I call on it most often for. That action is as a powerful anti-inflammatory and pain-relieving agent. There is a group of chemicals in ginger called *gingerols* that are known to give the anti-inflammatory action. This is because they interfere with an enzyme called *cyclo-oxygenase* (*COX*) that is involved in switching on inflammation and instigating pain. By blocking these enzymes, gingerols are able to prevent inflammation from occurring in the first place. Gingerols are also potent antioxidants, which can also help in the reduction of inflammation, because some inflammatory processes involve the release of free radicals. Free radicals are highly reactive biochemicals that cause all manner of damage and chaos in the body. Antioxidants are nutrients and plant chemicals that can deactivate the mischievous free radicals and protect body tissues from their destructive actions.

▶ **Best way to use**
As a juice, or added liberally to cooked dishes.

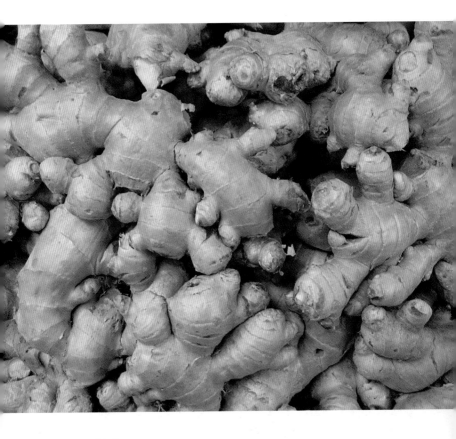

Horseradish

This staple of the British Sunday roast is actually a close relative of the cabbage. It has a long history of use in European herbal medicine. The leaves used to be a traditional salad vegetable, but it is the root that has given horseradish its reputation.

Horseradish contains a cocktail of volatile chemicals, including compounds such as myrosinase, that all react together to give it its mustard-like flavour. It is this cocktail of chemicals that give rise to its most famous of uses – as a remedy for sinusitis. The mustard-like chemistry can rapidly thin mucous and reduce inflammation while stimulating circulation.

Horseradish has also been traditionally used as a cholagogue, which means that it helps to increase the flow of bile from the gall bladder. This gives it a number of benefits. Firstly, it means that the liver is able to remove broken down toxins faster. Our liver uses bile as a transport medium to carry away any toxins that aren't water-soluble and can't be flushed out via the kidneys. The bile carries these toxins into the intestine for removal via the bowel. Secondly, horseradish was also traditionally used as a potent diuretic, meaning that it helped to increase urinary flow. It was mixed with cider vinegar and honey, and taken in drop dosages throughout the day.

▶ **Best way to use**

Ideally, the grated fresh root should be used. However, this is extremely strong, so may not suit everyone. Also, availability may be an issue. If fresh isn't available, then a high quality horseradish sauce will give equally impressive results.

Marjoram (Oregano)

Marjoram is a type of oregano. It is a staple herb in both Greek and Italian cooking. It has also been used medicinally for centuries.

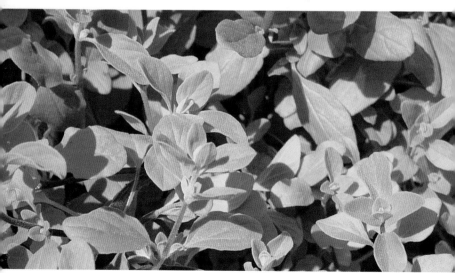

It contains two strong aromatic oils – thymol and carvacrol, which are believed to be responsible for the antimicrobial and natural antibiotic activity of marjoram. It has been traditionally used for food poisoning, amoebic dysentery, and other digestive upsets.

Marjoram is also an effective carminative, meaning it helps to break down gas within the digestive tract, to reduce bloating and flatulence.

▶ **Best way to use**
Fresh is key. I find it heavenly added to dishes such as roasted vegetables, and ratatouille. For relief of gas and bloating, I'd advise making a strong tea from the fresh leaves, and sipping slowly.

Mint

Mint has to be one of the most widely known and widely used herbs. It has a history of culinary and medicinal use in every conceivable culture, throughout all recorded periods of history, and it is a common feature in many gardens, parks, and wild open spaces. It is a native plant to the Mediterranean, and has found itself part of traditions stemming from ancient Greece, and ancient Rome. It was the Romans that gave us the ever popular mint sauce that finds itself onto many a Sunday dinner table.

Mint is a wonderful remedy for any kind of digestive discomfort. It is high in the essential oils 'carvacrol', 'thymol', and 'menthol' (the oil responsible for the unmistakable smell of mint). These powerful oils are highly effective carminatives, helping to break down and remove gas and wind from the digestive tract. The essential oils found in mint are also very effective antispasmodics. This means that they help to relax the muscles that line the walls of the digestive tract. This is useful for conditions such as irritable bowel syndrome and nervous diarrhoea.

Mint has also been traditionally used in cough and cold formulae. This is because the menthol content of mint has a reputation for "tightening" up the mucous membranes, helping to dry up excessive mucous during a cold. Menthol is also thought to be a diaphoretic, meaning that it encourages fever, thus helping to speed up infection recovery time.

▶ **Best way to use**

Fresh is generally better. It is an easy plant to grow in a pot at home, so that it is always on hand when we need it. For digestive problems, a tea made by infusing the fresh leaves in boiled water for 15–20 minutes is delicious and effective. Can also be eaten whole in any dish you fancy.

Mustard Seed

Mustard is a member of the cruciferous family of vegetables. This botanical family also includes broccoli, Brussels sprouts, and cabbage. There are several different types, but the one most commonly used is white mustard the type that makes the typical yellow English mustard condiment, that so many of us know and love. The ancient Romans are believed to be the first to experiment with various ways of preparing mustard seeds in a variety of culinary contexts. The most well documented was the mixing of crushed mustard seeds with an unfermented grape juice, commonly known in that period as "must". This combination made a preparation that was nicknamed "burning must", or in the language of that period "Mustum ardens". Hence the word "mustard" was born.

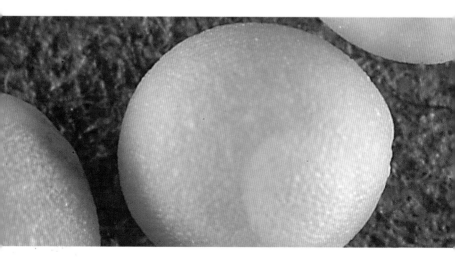

Mustard has been used medicinally since that period. The seeds are commonly used as a circulatory stimulant. The powerful essential oils that give mustard the distinctive fiery flavour can, like chilli peppers, cause a sudden and notable relaxation of the muscles within the blood vessel walls. Mustard has also been traditionally used as a poultice, applied directly onto the chest to help relieve a chesty cough.

▶ **Best way to use**
Use the seeds in curries, or a good quality fresh mustard, for a warming winter supplement, or to loosen mucous.

Parsley

Parsley has almost become a bit of a cliché in the culinary world. For years, it was the stereotypical herb used to decorate and garnish dishes, sprinkled haphazardly around the plate. It is also a classic ingredient in sauces for fish.

Parsley is a very powerful diuretic. It contains a strong essential oil (responsible for its fragrance and flavour), that acts as a very mild irritant to the filtration system in the kidney – the nephron. This irritation is harmless, yet notable enough to cause the kidney to increase the volume of urine that passes through at any one time. This makes parsley a great food to consider in cases of water retention. It should be avoided completely, however, if you have, or have recently had, a kidney infection or have any history of kidney disease.

▶ **Best way to use**
Use fresh in a salad, or as a fragrant, earthy tea.

Pepper

It's a fair assumption that pepper is on almost every table or in every kitchen in the UK and US. It has become a universal seasoning. This everyday addition to food gives us a little bit of an indication as to the way in which pepper was traditionally used as a medicine.

Pepper has long had a reputation of being a digestive aid. It is said to increase the force and regularity of peristaltic contractions (the rhythmical contractions that move gut contents along), and stimulate appetite. In Ayurveda, the traditional medical system of India, pepper is one of the favourite spices used to invigorate digestion, stimulate appetite, and to treat nausea. Pepper has such a powerful stimulatory, almost irritant, effect upon the digestive tract, that some patients awaiting abdominal surgery are advised not to consume it.

Pepper is also a diaphoretic, so is useful for encouraging a fever, which can help to reduce recovery time, when fighting an infection.

▶ **Best way to use**
Pepper can be incorporated into a herbal tea blend (use of pure pepper tea is not advisable), or added directly to food. In cases of weak digestion and poor appetite, a teaspoonful of ground black pepper can be taken, and washed down with a small glass of water.

Rosemary

Rosemary is without doubt one of the most commonly used, sold, and grown herbs in the UK. It is a very vigorous plant, which can take over a herb garden very easily if not kept in check. It is a native to the Mediterranean, and has been a part of Greek culture for centuries.

In Greece, it was traditionally used to enhance and to stimulate memory. This use still holds strong today, and rosemary is one of the most commonly used herbs in Western medical herbalism, for forgetfulness and a fuzzy head. Rosemary has this property due to its essential oil content. These powerful oils, like many of the culinary herbs, cause a widening of the blood vessels. This enhancement of circulation improves blood flow to the brain, and hence is believed to be the reason why rosemary delivers such improvements to memory. Rosemary, for the reasons outlined above, is also a common herb of choice for enhancing circulation in general. Any conditions such as cold fingers and toes will benefit greatly from the regular consumption of rosemary.

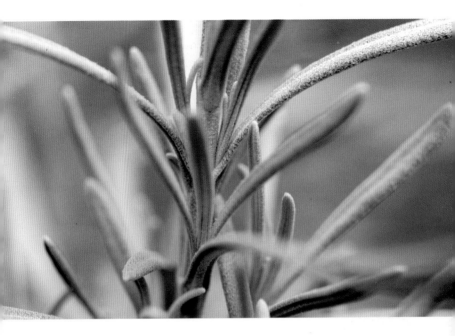

Rosemary has also become a popular anti-inflammatory herb of late. It contains a very powerful antioxidant compound called *rosmaric acid*. Some encouraging recent trials have suggested that rosmaric acid is able to combat inflammation, by causing a localized reduction in some of the chemicals that encourage inflammation.

Rosemary is also antispasmodic (helps to calm digestive cramps), and a diuretic.

▶ **Best way to use**
As a tea, or added fresh (don't overcook or process) to meals such as roasted vegetables, breads, potato dishes, etc.

Sage

Sage is another of our most widely known and widely used herbs. A staple of British cuisine, sage finds itself on many a Sunday dinner plate. Who can resist some sage and onion stuffing? Sage is viewed as a sacred plant in many cultures. It has been used in blessing ceremonies by Catholic priests, Native Americans, and some South American cultures. It is also often used for "smudging". This is the burning of sage, that has been tied up in a bundle, to "clear the energy" of a room or space.

Sage has gained the reputation of being an effective remedy for hot flushes associated with the menopause. It is often recommended to be used as a tea, while experiencing a hot flush. It is not entirely clear how sage does this, but its anecdotal track record is rather impressive. It is also believed to be antihidrotic, meaning it reduces perspiration. It is also believed to reduce lactation, so any pregnant or breastfeeding women should avoid consuming sage in high amounts.

Sage is also a renowned antibiotic agent. It contains powerful fragrant essential oils that seem to be very good at killing harmful oral bacteria. This is why sage has been a popular ingredient in herbal mouthwashes and breath fresheners. Many people believe that this was one of the major reasons that sage was originally included in many meat-based recipes – to help destroy any harmful bacteria that may be in the food. It was also used as a compress, applied directly to wounds, to minimize the risk of infection.

Sage is also believed to be a stimulant, general tonic, and memory aid.

▶ **Best way to use**
As with many of the herbs and spices, fresh is always the best. Take as a strong tea for hot flushes, or incorporate into salads or cooked dishes for its general tonic properties.

Thyme

Another of the classics, thyme is one of the true garden heroes. It is another Mediterranean staple that has become quite common in British cuisine. Frequently used in casseroles, breads, on pizzas, and in many meat-based dishes.

Thyme is also an old faithful, staple ingredient in any herbalist's medicine cabinet. It is very high in three exceptionally powerful essential oils – borneol, geraniol, and thymol. These potent oils give thyme its renowned antibacterial properties. Thyme is traditionally used as a gargle, and seems to be particularly effective at treating strep throat infections and tonsillitis. When used topically, thyme is also a potent antifungal.

The most interesting thing about thyme, in my opinion, is the evidence emerging that thyme may be highly beneficial for the health of the brain. Early studies suggest that something in thyme's chemistry enables it to increase the levels of a certain fat, called *DHA*, into cell membranes. DHA is something that is created in our bodies from dietary omega 3, from sources such as nuts, seeds, and avocados. It is used to maintain the structure of cells and tissues, and is most widely found in nerve cells. In our brain and nervous system, the cells have a very unique and specialized structure. They have large, elongated, fatty capsules along their entire length. These capsules do not touch, however. There is a tiny gap between the point where one capsule

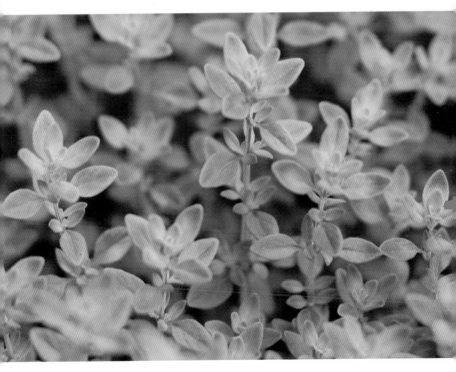

ends and the next starts. As you may know, each cell in the brain and nervous system communicates with the next via electrical signals. To make these signals travel at high speed, the cell allows the electrical signal to jump along the cell surface, using these little "unexposed" areas between capsules. The fatty substance DHA is vital for keeping the structure and function of this system in check. Therefore, by ensuring that we have healthy levels of DHA in the cells, we can help these cells to work to their optimal potential, and it is here that the consumption of thyme looks most promising.

▶ **Best way to use**
Use either fresh or dried. The secret is to add it to dishes at a fairly late stage where possible. This will deliver flavour without damaging too much of the active chemistry.

Turmeric

Turmeric, the staple ingredient of Indian curries, is in the same family as ginger, and shares some of its properties. It is a knobbly brown root, with vivid orange flesh, and a zingy invigorating aroma. Turmeric has been used in traditional Indian Ayurvedic herbal practices for centuries, and has even made its way into cosmetic products.

Like ginger, turmeric is a powerful anti-inflammatory agent. The chemicals that give turmeric its distinctive vibrant yellow/orange colour are key to its powerful inflammation-busting activity. These are a chemical group known as curcuminoids. The anti-inflammatory activity of these compounds has, in clinical trials, been shown to be comparable to such powerful drugs as hydrocortisone, phenylbutazone, indomethacin, and Nurofen. These amazing compounds reduce inflammation, by blocking the activity of a group of chemical messengers called *prostaglandins*. You may recall from previous sections of this book that prostaglandins are a group of chemical compounds made in the body from dietary fats. Part of their physiological role is to regulate the inflammatory response. This involves a series of chemical reactions that finally lead to a localized inflammatory response. Curcuminoids from turmeric block the normal progress of these chemical reactions and prevent them from reaching their goal.

Turmeric is also a great spice for the health of the heart and cardiovascular system. It is what herbalists refer to as "anti-platelet". Platelets are small, disk-like cells within the blood that are involved in the formation of blood clots, and are the agents at play when a scab forms. Clotting is a vital process that protects us from bleeding to death from the smallest of cuts, and allows us to heal internal injuries rapidly. However, it is problematic when we clot excessively, as this, along with other active risk factors, puts us at greater risk of heart attack and stroke. Turmeric helps to reduce the platelets' clotting capacity – not to the extent that it becomes dangerous, but enough to offer that little bit of extra protection against heart attacks.

Turmeric is also believed to be "hepato-protective". This means that it may help protect the liver from damage. The bright orange pigments, the curcuminoids, are also very powerful antioxidants. This is the most likely reason why turmeric offers this protection to the liver.

► **Best way to use**
If you can find the fresh root, then that's fantastic. You could use it grated or finely chopped. Chances are though that you will find it as a powder. Add this at any stage of cooking to curries, savoury dips, stews, soups, etc.

Vegetables

I think it is fair to say that nothing else has forged the same love/hate relationship as the humble vegetable. Once the absolute staple of our diet, vegetables are now becoming consumed on an alarmingly reduced scale. I have first-hand experience of working with people under the age of twenty, who had no idea what simple ingredients like beetroot, sweet potatoes, and courgettes were. This seems to be very representative of modern dietary trends – a trend that can, and most likely will, deliver severe health consequences in future generations.

The term vegetable isn't actually a specific scientific or botanical term in any way. It is generally meant to describe an edible plant, or a plant with edible portions, that doesn't come into the botanical class of fruit or seed. However, that is as far as the distinctions go, so the term can often be rather arbitrary. Some may consider mushrooms and avocados vegetables, whereas others may not. It all gets a bit fuzzy.

Vegetables are most likely the most suitable foods for human consumption, above all other food categories, and certainly offer some of the most powerful, profound, and complex medicinal activities found in the plant kingdom. Some have powerful colour pigments that can offer protection against chemical damage, or even speed up or slow down certain functions. Some deliver their medicinal activity via their complex flavours, while some offer us therapeutic benefit through the action of chemicals that they produce naturally during normal growth.

This is just one of a million arguments for making the main proportion of our diet plant-based.

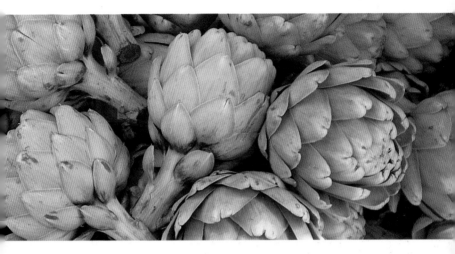

(Globe) Artichoke

Globe artichoke is actually a type of thistle, and is probably one of those vegetables that you have always seen on the supermarket shelves, and thought... hmm... looks nice, but I have no idea what to do with it! This unusual-looking vegetable is actually an unopened edible flower. The outer leaves are very tough and inedible, but the central flesh (hearts) is absolutely heavenly to eat.

Globe artichoke contains a group of chemicals called *caffeoylquinic acids*. These compounds are responsible for artichoke's traditional usage for liver disorders. Artichoke comes into the herbal category that herbalists call cholerectic. This means that it increases the flow of bile from the liver. This is important because the liver uses bile as a transport medium for toxins that it has broken down, that need removing from the body. Bile is also involved in the digestion and absorption of fat, so eating artichoke alongside a fatty meal aids digestion. It is also believed that artichoke may also be able to lower cholesterol by having an impact on the way in which cholesterol is broken down in the liver. The cholesterol-lowering effect may also be due to artichoke's ability to speed up the movement of fatty material (which is the material used to make cholesterol) out of the liver.

Artichoke is also believed to be an ideal diabetic food. This is because it is high in a special kind of sugar known as inulin. Inulin is believed to play a beneficial role in blood sugar management, helping other sugars consumed alongside it to be released into the bloodstream at a far slower pace.

▶ **Best way to use**
Lightly roasted, or baked. As fresh as possible.

Asparagus

I love asparagus, especially lightly steamed with a little melted butter and black pepper. Heaven! Luckily, it is a very nutrient dense and medicinal vegetable, not to mention the slightly luxurious associations it has.

Asparagus has proved to be a very effective diuretic agent – meaning it will increase urinary output. This is thanks to a nitrogenous compound called *asparagine*. This is why asparagus has

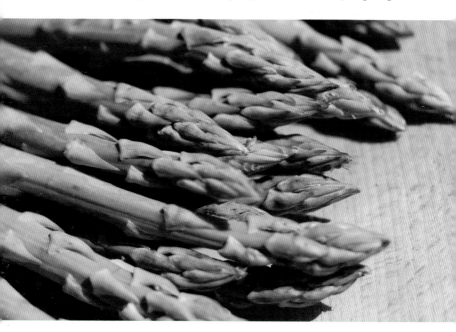

been used in traditional medicine as a tonic for kidney health and for fluid retention. If kidney output is stimulated, then a far more rapid removal of excessive fluids in the body will ensue. This stimulation will also give the kidneys a bit of a flush too, helping to remove metabolic waste and debris.

Asparagus is also showing some potential as an anti-inflammatory food. It contains a powerful phytochemical called *racemofuran*, which is believed to work in a similar way to a group of pharmaceutical anti-inflammatory drugs called *COX-2 inhibitors*. This means that it can actually partially block the series of chemical chain reactions that arise when the inflammatory response is activated.

Some members of the asparagus family have been used for centuries in traditional Indian Ayurvedic medicine to increase fertility and to regulate the menstrual cycle. It is believed by many that the regular, culinary asparagus has the same properties. There is little phytochemical data available at present that supports this, however.

▶ **Best way to use**
Steam, or sauté. Do NOT boil!

Aubergine

I love these Mediterranean delights. They are just like big sponges that will suck up almost any flavour that is added to them.

Aubergine has often been seen as having little in the way of nutrition, or major health benefit, apart from being a good source of dietary fibre. However, in recent years, a compound called *nasunin* was discovered in the skin of aubergine. Nasunin has been shown to protect the fatty membranes of cells within the nervous system and brain from chemical damage. Scientists now believe that long-term consumption may offer some protection against degenerative mental disorders such as dementia.

▶ **Best way to use**
Lightly cooked, roasted and puréed to make baba ganoush.

Beetroot (Beet)

Beetroot has to be one of my absolute favourite vegetables ever. There is nothing quite like big chunks of slow-roasted beetroot, with horseradish sauce, as an accompaniment to my Sunday lunch. It is in the same family as spinach and chard, and comes in many different varieties, with colours ranging from white, through to vivid golden yellow. For our purposes here, however, we will focus upon the common, deep purple variety.

The deep purple pigment, that gives beetroot its characteristic colour, that stains almost anything it touches, is part of the key to beetroot's medicinal properties. This vivid colour pigment is a compound called *betacyanin*. Betacyanin has been shown to increase certain chemical functions in the liver that form part of what is known as "phase 2 detoxification". It essentially speeds up certain chemical reactions that are involved in the smooth running of this process. Phase 2 detoxification is one of the series of processes that the liver uses to turn harmful toxins, such as alcohol and metabolic wastes, into harmless substances that can easily be removed from the body. This makes beetroot a useful food for detoxification and liver-cleansing.

Beetroot is also known to have a very beneficial effect upon blood pressure. It contains a chemical called *nitrate*. When we consume nitrate, it gets converted by the body into a compound called *nitric oxide*. Nitric oxide is a powerful vasodilator (widens blood vessels). It does this by forcing a sudden relaxation of the muscular walls that line the blood vessels. When these muscles relax, the internal size of the vessel increases, so, therefore, the pressure within the vessel naturally decreases.

Beetroot is also believed to be a powerful anti-cancer food. This is because it increases the production of one of the body's own "anti-cancer chemicals", produced to protect cells from damage. This protective chemical is a compound called glutathione-s-transferase.

▶ **Best way to use**
Juiced, grated raw, or roasted in big chunks.

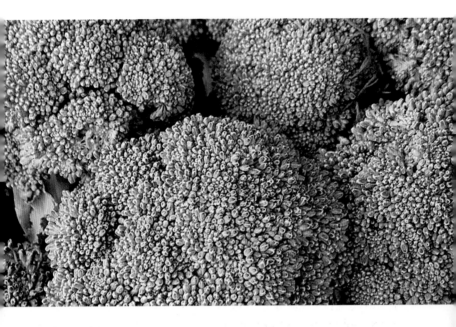

Broccoli

Broccoli, like cabbage and cauliflower, is a member of the cruciferous vegetable family. Unlike most of the ingredients discussed in this book, broccoli doesn't have a fast-acting medicinal effect. It does, however, have some very powerful disease-preventing properties that warrant its discussion.

Broccoli is probably the most highly regarded food for cancer prevention. This is due to the high levels of three powerful cancer-fighting phytochemical groups – isothiocyanates, indoles, and dithiolethiones. These almost unpronounceable chemicals protect the body from cancer by regulating the way in which cells respond to environmental elements that can potentially trigger cancerous changes within the DNA of the cell. They do this by increasing the cell's natural defence mechanisms against damage, making it more resistant.

▶ **Best way to use**
As fresh as possible. Steamed, stir fried, or raw.

Cabbage

Without doubt, our most abundant and affordable green vegetable, and one of the most powerful foods you can include in your weekly diet. Better still, they are easy to grow, and it won't take long to have your own supply of fresh, locally grown, super greens.

Cabbages, like all of the brassicas, contain a whole cocktail of phytochemicals that can have a huge impact upon normal detoxification of the cells in all of our tissues. They do this by interacting with the control centre for each cell – its DNA. They communicate a message that encourages the cell's DNA to produce more enzymes within the cell that actually enable and facilitate the normal detoxification and breakdown of potentially harmful toxic material.

Cabbages are also a rich source of phytochemicals such as indole-3-carbinol and isothiocyanates, which have potent anti-cancer properties.

There is also a link between cabbage consumption and lowered risk of heart disease. This is because cabbage has a strong ability to lower a compound called *homocysteine*, which is believed to be one of the biggest risk factors for heart disease. It is not entirely clear whether homocysteine itself plays a functional role in the development of heart disease, or whether its presence is just an indicator of other risks. What is clear is that lowering elevated levels certainly does reduce one's heart attack risk.

▶ **Best way to use**
Steamed, sautéed, or raw. Boiled cabbage is of no great use to man or beast, unless of course creating noxious odours in your kitchen serves a practical use. Boiling this precious vegetable will make it devoid of any of the good stuff.

Carrots

These bright orange vegetable staples are among our most commonly consumed vegetables, although quite often we find them boiled to the point of semi-existence, alongside a few manky peas. However, carrots can be incredibly powerful both nutritionally and medicinally.

The bright orange colour of carrots is due to the massive concentration of the plant source of vitamin A, called *beta carotene*. This chemical is a colour pigment from the carotenoid group, responsible for colours ranging between pale yellow to deep dark red in the plant kingdom. Beta carotene is known to be highly protective of the heart and cardiovascular system, by helping to protect the structural integrity of the inner lining of the blood vessels, thus helping to reduce rupture and injury that can lead to the formation of clots.

Beta carotene is also famous for improving eye health. Firstly, it improves night vision, hence the old wives' tale "carrots help you see in the dark". Secondly, it is known to protect an area of the eye known as the macula densa; the area that falls victim to macular degeneration. This age-associated damage to the eye is caused by the activity of free radicals. Beta carotene has an affinity with this tissue, and is extremely good at disarming this type of free radical.

▶ **Best way to use**
Raw, grated in salads, or as a crudité with a dip such as hummus. This combination is especially good, as the fats in the hummus will help the beta carotene to be absorbed faster.

Celery

This stringy salad staple may seem like the most innocuous food in the world. It is definitely one of those foods that people either love or hate, and sometimes getting it down many of my clients can be a real challenge. This food that we all imagine to be dull and useless is, in fact, a very powerful medicinal food.

Celery contains a powerful compound called *3-N-Butylphthalide* (3NB for short), which is a powerful painkiller. I have found it to be useful in cases of arthritis, sprains, and many issues involving chronic pain. Its effect isn't hugely long-lasting, like taking a prescription painkiller, but it is a beautiful example of the type of simple food that can be incorporated into one's daily routine, that can assist in overall healing and comfort.

Celery also contains a fragrant group of chemicals called *coumarins*. These are part of the chemistry that give celery its distinct smell, and are also the same chemicals that fill the air when a lawn is being mown. Coumarins are amazing at ridding body tissues of any build-ups of fluid. They help to stimulate the lymphatic system, which is the main system that drains and clears waste and gunk that is released from the tissues. Coumarins help to increase uptake of excessive fluids by the lymphatic system. Coumarins also have a mild diuretic property, which further support their ability to remove excess fluid from the body. This makes celery an ideal food for cycle-related fluid retention, arthritis (removes fluid build-up from joints), and can even help with the lowering of blood pressure.

▶ **Best way to use**

Eaten raw or juiced. Cooked celery is completely useless as even the slightest heat exposure can break down its active constituents, leaving it with not much else to offer.

Fennel

Fennel is another of those vegetables that many people seem to see on the supermarket shelf, pick up with a semi-bewildered expression, and then put back and move on. It is definitely overlooked. This is unfortunate, because fennel has some wonderful health-giving properties, and it is such an easy vegetable to prepare, and gives a glorious flavour.

Fennel contains a very powerful and beautifully fragrant essential oil called *anethol*. Anethol has been shown to be a very powerful anti-inflammatory. It delivers this activity, by reducing the amount of certain chemical signals released by some white blood cells that encourage localized inflammation. Anethol is also the main chemical responsible for fennel's famous antispasmodic effects. This means it helps to reduce and regulate normal contractions of the gut wall. This makes fennel useful in cases of painful abdominal cramps and IBS. The essential oils in fennel are also carminative, meaning they help to reduce and disperse gas from the digestive tract.

Fennel is also relatively high in phyto-oestrogens. These are plant chemicals that are similar in chemical structure to the female hormone oestrogen. These compounds are known to be of great use in any type of condition where a change in oestrogen levels is causing symptoms, such as menopause and pre menstrual issues. In cases where oestrogen levels are very low, it is believed that phyto-oestrogens are able to make the body think that there is more oestrogen available than there really is. In cases where oestrogen is too high, it is believed that phyto-oestrogens can actually compete against natural oestrogen, for binding sites on the outer surfaces of cells, thus reducing oestrogen's impact.

▶ **Best way to use**
Sliced raw, or lightly roasted. The fine top foliage can be chopped and eaten raw.

Kale

Kale has easily got to be one of my favourite foods. It is so juicy, green, delicious, and divine. It is wholesome and filling and leaves me feeling wonderful after I have eaten it.

Kale is proving to be an especially useful food for those with high cholesterol. This is because it contains a chemical called *indole-3-carbinol*. This miraculous compound actually reduces the production of

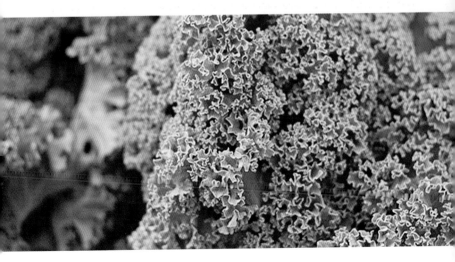

a cholesterol-carrying molecule called *apolipoproteinB-100*. This is one of the main transporter chemicals involved in carrying cholesterol away from the liver to the other tissues in the body, which may lead to a harmful build-up. Indole-3-carbinol reduces this cholesterol by around 56 per cent. This clever compound also seems to have an impact on the extent to which the liver manufactures blood lipids (fats), which can lead to elevated cholesterol.

Kale, like any of the brassicas, contains a very high level of sulphur-based compounds, including glucosinolates, which help to increase cells' ability to process and break down potentially cancerous chemicals. There is a long accepted link between the consumption of cruciferous vegetables and reduced risk of cancers. This is most likely the reason why.

▶ **Best way to use**
Delicious eaten raw. Drizzle with olive oil and a pinch of salt, and massage to wilt the leaves. If you cook it, steam it lightly, or stir fry quickly.

Leeks

I never used to like leeks particularly, but now I just can't get enough of them. Every Sunday, I have leeks with butter and black pepper as a side accompaniment to my Sunday lunch, week in, week out.

Leeks, like all of the alliums, are very high in sulphur-based compounds such as allicin that can help to reduce clotting in the blood, and can give a notable antiviral effect. These compounds also play a role in naturally lowering cholesterol, and protect from certain cancers.

There is another interesting cancer-fighting phytochemical that is found in leeks. That is a compound called *kaempferol*. A well known Nurses' Health Study, that ran between 1984 and 2002, revealed that women with the highest intake of kaempferol had a 40 per cent reduction in the risk of developing ovarian cancer. While this observational study hasn't been backed up by further clinical data, it certainly gives some interesting information about the potential properties of this often underrated allium.

▶ **Best way to use**
Any really. I have a preference for sautéing it in olive oil and butter, with a good pinch of sea salt and black pepper. Also great in soups.

Onions

One of the kings of the vegetable kingdom without a shadow of a doubt. I use them in nearly every savoury dish that I make. I especially love red onions. The gorgeous red/purple pigment delivers higher levels of antioxidants than the white counterparts.

Onions are a very rich source of an antioxidant compound called *quercetin*, which is a very effective natural antihistamine. Histamine is a chemical that is released locally by white blood cells when they are exposed to certain stimuli that cause allergic type symptoms. It is this localized histamine release that causes symptoms such as itching, sneezing, inflammation, etc, that we associate with allergy. Quercetin appears to be very effective at reducing the ability of these cells to release their histamine when stimulated.

Onions are also believed to be potent anti-inflammatories – especially for the respiratory tract. They contain compounds that have been shown to inhibit the effect of specific communication chemicals that increase the production of pro-inflammatory prostaglandins (see the Joints section). These body chemicals, called *lipoxygenase* and *cyclooxygenase*, are substances that actually cause a drastic shift in the production of these problematic inflammatory stimulants, so any natural substances that can reduce this from occurring can have a massive impact upon the severity and duration of inflammatory episodes. Granted, onions aren't as powerful as taking a high strength drug, but like foods such as ginger and turmeric, they are an ideal food for helping to deliver an overall reduction in inflammation.

Onions are also a wonderful food for overall digestive health. They contain a fabulous compound called *inulin* that works as a prebiotic agent. This means that it encourages the growth of good bacteria in the gut, by providing them with a food source. This helps to increase the numbers of the good, and decrease the number of the bad, fine-tuning digestive health when consumed regularly.

▶ **Best way to use**
Raw or lightly sautéed.

Peppers

These crunchy salad vegetables pack quite a powerful punch, both medicinally and nutritionally. From the nutritional perspective, they are very high in vitamin C, some of the B vitamins, and also vitamin A.

Peppers, especially the red ones, are very dense in compounds called *carotenoids*. These are colour pigments in plants that can range from yellows, to oranges, to reds. These powerful pigments have a strong antioxidant activity and have been linked with increased protection against cancers. They are also believed to play a role in slowing down age-related damage to the eyes, and offer protection against cataracts.

▶ **Best way to use**
Raw or very lightly stir fried or sautéed.

Potatoes

Once considered the dieter's "enemy", these starchy staples are going through something of a renaissance. I have to admit, I never ate them often, but now Sundays and roast potatoes are a symbiotic relationship in my eyes! And now that new research has revealed some amazing chemical properties, I can eat these almost guilt free!

New research has identified a compound in potatoes called *kukoamine*. This rare compound is found in some Chinese herbs, and nobody thought for a second that it may turn up in the humble spud! Kukoamine has actually been shown to lower blood pressure. Research is still in the very early days and, as such, nobody is entirely sure how kukoamine does this, or indeed how many potatoes need to be consumed in order to have a significant impact.

▶ **Best way to use**

Generally, steamed, boiled, or baked. Keep consumption of roasted/fried potatoes to a minimum... roasties are supposed to be a once a week treat after all.

Spinach

Popeye's famous staple food. Spinach is, without doubt, one of the most powerful foods on the planet. Firstly, it is a nutrient-packed powerhouse. It contains more usable protein gram for gram than a sirloin steak; more usable calcium than any dairy product, and a whole host of B vitamins.

More exciting than this, though, is the huge array of cancer-fighting compounds found in spinach. It contains a group of 13–14 flavonoid chemicals, collectively known as methylenedioxyflavonol glucuronides (try saying that one really fast!). These compounds have proved so powerful, that they have prompted myriads of clinical trials with spinach extracts. These trials have shown a high level of protection

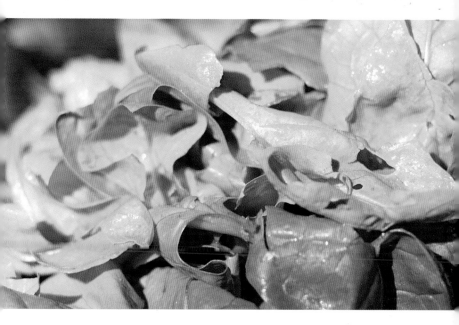

against cancers of the stomach, prostate, and the ovaries. The picture is especially interesting in the case of prostate cancer. One of the chemical fractions of the chemical group mentioned above is a compound called *neoxanthin*. This amazing phytochemical has been shown to force cancerous prostate cells into a state that is known as "apoptosis", which is the suicide state programmed into each and every cell in the body. When this function is stimulated, the cell dies in minutes. The fascinating story doesn't end there. When neoxanthin is being digested and processed in the intestines, a certain proportion of it will be converted into a substance called *neochromes*. These substances put cancerous prostate cells into a state of stasis, which helps to slow down any kind of major progression of the disease.

So what are you waiting for folks, get that spinach down you!

► **Best way to use**

Raw is absolutely the best way to consume spinach, and it makes the base of virtually all of my salads. You can also steam and sauté it. However, because many of the active compounds in spinach are water-soluble, boiling causes them to leach out into the water, which means that boiled spinach is about as much use as an ashtray on a motorbike, so forget that idea!

Sweet Potatoes

I absolutely love sweet potatoes. I love the colour, the texture, and the delicious sweet flavour. I tend to use them in curries and in soups too.

Sweet potatoes are a very dense and rich source of the potent antioxidant beta carotene. This is the compound responsible for sweet potatoes' characteristic, bright orange colour. Beta carotene is not only the plant form of vitamin A, it is also a powerful anti-inflammatory. This is mostly due to its antioxidant activity being able to buffer some of the nasty inflammatory activity delivered by white blood cells.

Sweet potatoes also contain a unique protein. This is a storage protein that the plant uses as a food source as it is growing. This fantastic protein is what is known as an immunomodulator, meaning it can help to regulate certain responses within the immune system.

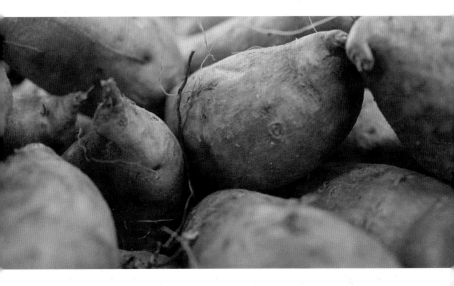

Again, much of the research regarding this activity is in its early stages. What we do know, however, is that it interacts with elements of the immune system that instigate and worsen the inflammatory response.

I also find sweet potatoes to be wonderful for digestive health. They contain a wonderful sugar called *fructo-oligo-saccharide* (*FOS*). This sugar is a prebiotic, meaning that it can actually encourage the growth of good bacteria in the gut. When the population of good bacteria in our digestive system feeds upon this sugar, they begin to reproduce, thus increasing the colony. That's not all. When the good bacteria feed upon FOS, they actually produce a chemical called *butyric acid* that can repair and strengthen the gut wall, helping to regenerate and rejuvenate the digestive tract.

Sweet potatoes are also believed to be very good for diabetics. It appears that they have an ability to help to stabilize blood sugar levels, and to improve cells' responsiveness to insulin. It isn't entirely clear what is responsible for this at present.

▶ **Best way to use**

I love them baked, in place of the traditional baked potato. They are also great in soups, curries, and roasted with garlic.

Index